Behavioral
Pharmacology

Behavioral Pharmacology

Susan D. Iversen
Department of Psychology
University of Cambridge

Leslie L. Iversen
Department of Pharmacology
University of Cambridge

1975
Oxford University Press
New York and Oxford

Acknowledgments

Figure 1-1. Figure 2. M. M. Shapiro, *J. exp. Anal. Behav.* 4, 361 (1961). Reprinted by permission of the Society for the Experimental Analysis of Behavior, Inc.

Figure 1-2. Figure 1. N. E. Miller and L. DiCara, *J. comp. physiol. Psychol.* 63, 12 (1967). Reprinted by permission of the authors. Copyright © 1967 by the American Psychological Association. Reprinted by permission of the publisher.

Figures 1-3, 1-5, 1-8. G. S. Reynolds, *A Primer of Operant Conditioning.* Copyright © 1968 by Scott, Foresman and Co. Reprinted by permission of the publisher and author.

Figure 1-4. Figure 1. R. T. Kelleher and W. H. Morse, *Ergebn. der Physiol.* 60, 1 (1968). Reprinted by permission of the authors and Springer-Verlag, Heidelberg.

Figures 1-6, 3-5, 4-2, 4-10, 4-11, 4-21. Figures 3, 4, 5, 6, 7, and 8. R. T. Kelleher and W. H. Morse, *Fed. Proc.* 23, 808 (1964). Reprinted with the permission of the authors. Copyright © 1964 by Federation of American Societies for Experimental Biology, Bethesda, Maryland.

Figure 1-7. Figure 2. E. Hearst, M. B. Koresko, and R. Poppen, *J. exp. Anal. Behav.* 7, 369 (1964). Reprinted by permission of the authors and the Society for the Experimental Analysis of Behavior, Inc.

Figure 1-9. Figure 1. J. W. McKearney, *Science* 160, 1249 (1968). Reprinted by permission of the author. Copyright © 1968 by the American Association for the Advancement of Science.

Figure 1-10. Figures 3, 4, and 5. N. H. Azrin, W. C. Holtz, and D. F. Hake, *J. exp. anal. Behav.* 6, 141 (1963). Reprinted by permission of the authors and the Society for the Experimental Analysis of Behavior, Inc.

Figure 1-11. Figure 1. H. F. Hunt, and J. W. Brady, *J. comp. physiol. Psychol.* 44, 88 (1951). Reprinted by permission of the authors. Copyright © 1951 by the American Psychological Association. Reprinted by permission of the publisher.

Acknowledgments

Figure 1-12. Figure, pp. 52-53. H. S. Liddell. Copyright © 1954 by Scientific American, Inc. All rights reserved.

Figure 1-13. Figure 1. N. H. Azrin, R. R. Hutchinson, and D. F. Hake, *J. exp. anal. Behav.* 9, 191 (1966). Reprinted by permission of the authors and the Society for the Experimental Analysis of Behavior, Inc.

Figure 1-14. Figure 1. R. R. Hutchinson, N. H. Azrin, and G. M. Hunt. *J. exp. anal. Behav.* 11, 489 (1968). Reprinted by permission of the authors and the Society for the Experimental Analysis of Behavior, Inc.

Figure 1-15. Figure 2. D. R. Cherek, T. Thompson, and G. T. Heistad, *J. exp. anal. Behav.* 19, 113 (1973). Reprinted by permission of the authors and the Society for the Experimental Analysis of Behavior, Inc.

Figures 2-1, 2-2. Figures 1-57 and 1-59. A. Goldstein, L. Aranow, and S. M. Kalman, *Principles of Drug Action.* Copyright © 1969 by Harper & Row, New York. Reprinted by permission of the authors and publisher.

Figure 2-3. Figure 1. K. M. Taylor and S. H. Snyder, *Brain Res.* 28, 295 (1971). Reprinted by permission of the authors and Elsevier Publishing Company, Amsterdam.

Figure 2-4. Figure 5. A. Goldstein and P. Sheehan, *J. Pharmac. exp. Ther.* 169, 175 (1969). Reprinted by permission of the authors. Copyright © 1964 by The Williams & Wilkins Co. Baltimore.

Figure 2-5. Figure 1, p. 65. A. Peters in *Contemporary Research Methods in Neuroanatomy,* eds. W. J. H. Nauta and S. O. E. Ebbesson (1970). Copyright © 1970 by Springer-Verlag, New York. Reprinted by permission of the author and publisher.

Figure 2-6. Figure 12, p. 11. G. D. Pappas and S. T. G. Waxman in *Structure and Function of Synapses,* eds. G. D. Pappas and D. D. Purpura. Copyright © 1972 by Raven Press, New York. Reprinted by permission of the authors and publisher.

Figures 2-7, 2-14. Figures 3 and 6, pp. 93 and 99. R. H. Rech and K. E. Moore, *An Introduction to Psychopharmacology.* Copyright © 1971 by Raven Press, New York. Reprinted by permission of the authors and publisher.

Figure 2-8. Figure 2. P. B. Bradley and J. Elkes, *Brain* 80, 77 (1957). Reprinted by permission of the authors and Macmillan Journals Ltd.

Figure 2-9. Figure 1. B. S. Bunney, G. K. Aghajanian, and R. H. Roth, *Nature (New Biology)* 245, 123 (1973). Reprinted by permission of the authors and Macmillan Journals Ltd.

Figure 2-11. Figure 1. J. S. Kelly and L. P. Renaud, *Brit. J. Pharmac.* 48, 369 (1973). Reprinted by permission of the authors and Macmillan Journals Ltd.

Figure 2-20. Figure 7. T. Hokfelt and A. Ljungdahl, *Histochemie* 29, 325 (1972). Reprinted by permission of the authors and Springer-Verlag, Heidelberg.

Acknowledgments

Figures 2-21, 2-22. Figures 3 and 4. B. Livett, *Brit. Med. Bull.* 29, 2 (1973). Reprinted by permission of the author and publisher, the Medical Department, The British Council, 65, Davies Street, London W.1.

Figure 2-24. Figure C. C. C. D. Shute and P. R. Lewis, *Brain* 99, 487 (1967). Reprinted by permission of the authors and Macmillan Journals Ltd.

Figure 3-1. Figure 4. P. B. Dews. *J. Pharmac. exp. Ther.* 113, 393 (1955). Reprinted by permission of the author and publisher. Copyright © 1955 by The Williams & Wilkins Co., Baltimore.

Figure 3-2. Figure 2. W. H. Morse in *First Habnemann Symposium on Psychosomatic Medicine.* Reprinted by permission of the author and publisher. Copyright © 1962 by Lea & Febiger, New York.

Figure 3-3. Figure 5. P. B. Dews, *J. Pharmac. exp. Ther.* 122, 137 (1958). Reproduced by permission of the author and publisher. Copyright © 1958 by The Williams & Wilkins Co., Baltimore.

Figure 3-4. Figure 8. L. Cook and R. T. Kelleher, *N. Y. Acad. Sci.* 96, 315 (1962). Reproduced by permission of the author and the publisher.

Figure 3-6. Figures 1, 2, and 3. P. B. Dews, *J. Pharmac. exp. Ther.* 115, 380 (1955). Reproduced by permission of the author and publisher. Copyright © 1955 by The Williams & Wilkins Co., Baltimore.

Figures 3-7, 3-8. Figures 4, 5, and 6. B. Weiss and V. G. Laties, *Fed. Proc.* 23, 801 (1964). Reproduced by permission of the authors and the publisher. Copyright © 1964 by Federation of American Societies for Experimental Biology, Bethesda, Maryland.

Figure 3-9. Figure 4. P. B. Dews, *N-S Arch. exp. Path. u. Pharmak.* 248, 296 (1964). Reproduced by permission of the author and publisher, Springer-Verlag, Heidelberg.

Figures 3-10, 3-11. Figures 3, 4, and 7. W. H. Morse, *Psychopharmacologia* (Berl.) 6, 286 (1964). Reproduced by permission of the author and publisher, Springer-Verlag, Heidelberg.

Figure 4-3. Figure 1. S. H. Barondes and H. D. Cohen, *Science,* 160, 556 (1968). Reproduced by permission of the authors and publisher. Copyright © 1968 by the American Association for the Advancement of Science.

Figure 4-5. Figures 2, 3, and 4. G. E. Vaillant, *J. Pharmac. exp. Ther.* 146, 377 (1964). Reproduced by permission of the author and publisher. Copyright © 1964 by The Williams & Wilkins Co., Baltimore.

Figures 4-6, 4-18. Figures 3, 4, and 5. G. Zbinden and L. O. Randall, *Adv. Pharm.* 5, 213 (1967). Reproduced by permission of the authors and publisher, Academic Press, Inc., New York.

Figures 4-8, 4-9. Figures 2 and 4. B. Weiss and V. G. Laties, *J. Pharmac.*

Acknowledgments

exp. Ther. 143, 169 (1964). Reproduced by permission of the authors and publisher. Copyright © 1964 by The Williams & Wilkins Co., Baltimore.

Figure 4-12. Figure 6. A. Goldstein and P. Sheehan, *J. Pharmac. exp. Ther.* 169, 175 (1969). Reproduced by permission of the authors and publisher. Copyright © 1969 by The Williams & Wilkins Co., Baltimore.

Figures 4-13, 4-14. Figures 6 and 7. D. E. McMillan and W. H. Morse, *J. Pharmac. exp. Ther.* 157, 175 (1967). Reproduced by permission of the authors and publisher. Copyright © 1967 by The Williams & Wilkins Co., Baltimore.

Figure 4-15. Figure 1. C. R. S. Schuster and J. H. Woods, *Int. J. Addictions,* 3, 223 (1968). Reproduced by permission of the authors and publisher, Marcel Dekker (Publishing), Inc., New York.

Figure 4-17. Figures 1 and 4. I. Geller, J. T. Kulak, and J. Seifter, *Psychopharmacologia* (Berl.), 3, 374 (1962). Reproduced by permission of the author and publisher, Springer-Verlag, Heidelberg.

Figure 4-24. Figure 2. P. Black, S. N. Cianci, P. Spyropoulas, and J. D. Maser in *Drugs and the Brain,* ed. P. Black. Copyright © 1969 by Johns Hopkins Press, Baltimore.

Figure 5-1. Figure 9. P. A. J. Janssen, C. J. E. Niemegeers, and K. H. L. Schellekens, *Arzneim-Forsch.* 15, 104 (1965). Reproduced by permission of the authors and publisher, Editio Cantor-K. G. Publishers, Aulendorf, Germany.

Figure 5-2. Figure 1. U. Ungerstedt, *Acta. physiol. Scand. Suppl.* 367 (1971) p. 73. Reproduced by permission of the author and the publisher, Acta Physiologica Scandinavica, Stockholm.

Figure 5-3. Figure 2. R. Stretch and G. J. Gerber, *Canad. J. Psychol.* 27, 168 (1973). Reproduced by permission of the authors and publisher, Canadian Psychological Association.

Preface

Neuropharmacology is concerned with the study of the effects of drugs on nervous tissue; psychopharmacology is concerned with the study of the effects of drugs on behavior. The discovery, in recent years, of highly effective drugs for treating various categories of mental illness in man has stimulated research in both areas and encouraged closer ties between them. In several instances, these drugs are now known to have specific neuropharmacological actions, and this has provided an added impetus to efforts to define the effects of such drugs on normal animal behavior precisely and to devise animal model behavior systems for discovering and assessing modifications of these clinically valuable drugs.

In this book we describe the achievements of psychopharmacology in providing behavioral methods for assaying drug action, and we give a brief resumé of the subject matter of neuropharmacology. The major classes of psychoactive drugs are described from both of these points of view. In the final section, examples are described where the marriage of neuro- and psychopharmacology is throwing new light on some old clinical problems.

Cambridge   S.D.I.
January 1975   L.L.I.

Contents

Contents

Contents

Contents

Behavioral Pharmacology

1 | The Analysis of Behavior

There are many ways of studying behavior, and opinions differ as to which are the most useful assays for assessing pharmacological effects. In this chapter we will confess ourselves immediately to be advocates of the descriptive behaviorism originally expounded by B. F. Skinner. This approach is grounded in the belief that by selecting a clearly defined element of behavior and objectively describing its occurrence under a variety of conditions, a predictive explanation of behavior emerges. This approach avoids any subjective and anthropomorphic interpretations of animal behavior. Many have found such an approach to behavior unacceptable. Lever pressing in the rat or key pecking in the pigeon are viewed both as unnatural behaviors and as artificially selected elements of a much more complex behavior pattern. The relevance of studies of animal behavior to an understanding of human behavior, whether normal or abnormal, appears to reinforce the conviction that we should be concerned with "whole" behavior patterns rather than their individual elements. As Dews (1958) remarked, "why is it, that when somebody learns how to study a single nerve cell or a single renal tubule or to isolate a single enzyme everyone (rightly) says 'Bravo'; but when attempts are made to isolate functional units of behaviour for study many people say 'Ah, but you are neglecting all other concurrent behaviour and therefore your results are meaningless.'"

We hope to show, however, that the methods devised by

3

Skinner have served psychopharmacology well. In Chapter 1 the variables that determine patterns of responding are described, and in Chapters 3 and 4 we go on to show how the major classes of psychoactive drugs can be identified by the manner in which they modify the control these variables have over behavior.

NORMAL BEHAVIOR

Classical and operant conditioning

In this chapter we will review some of the principles and techniques used in the experimental analysis of animal behavior. Under natural conditions, an animal is observed to make two kinds of behavioral responses, ELICITED and EMITTED. ELICITED RESPONSES are those that can be induced reliably by a specific stimulus and under normal conditions only by that stimulus or one very similar to it. Such responses are reflexive; for example, withdrawal of a limb to a painful stimulus, pricking of the ear to sound, contraction of the pupil to light, and salivation to food. Elicited responses are precisely determined by the properties of the eliciting stimulus (its frequency of presentation, duration, and intensity) and are objectively quantified by their latency of onset, their amplitude, and the intensity of eliciting stimulus required to induce them. EMITTED RESPONSES, by contrast, are not induced by any identifiable stimulus. Rats, for example, placed in an activity box run about. The amount of running characteristically decreases gradually with time, and many variables, such as time of day, degree of deprivation, estrous state in the female, temperature, and experience with the box, influence the characteristics of this habituation. Yet in such situations, eliciting stimuli are not readily identified, and the behavior cannot therefore be controlled. If one is interested in using base lines of spontaneously emitted behavior for evaluating drug actions, one must resort to the observational methods of the ethologist, recording all the elements of behavior, as far as they can be defined, and their sequence. The studies of Chance and Silverman (1964) on rat social behavior provide an example of this method.

In certain natural patterns of behavior the relationship between emitted and elicited responses is complex. In many animals, for example, courtship and mating involves predominantly emitted behavior initially. Gradually, however, elicited behaviors under precise stimulus control emerge in sequence, and, finally, copulation, a reflexive action controlled primarily by the autonomic nervous system, occurs.

Elicited and emitted responses may be modified by conditioning. There are two kinds of conditioning—CLASSICAL (respondent or type 1) and OPERANT (instrumental or type 2)—and it is generally accepted that elicited responses are most easily conditioned classically and emitted responses operantly. Classical conditioning was originally described by Pavlov and is a process of stimulus substitution achieved by stimulus contiguity. A given response (the unconditioned response, UR) is elicited by a certain stimulus (unconditioned stimulus, US). A neutral stimulus (conditioned stimulus, CS) that would not normally elicit the response (UR) is presented at the same time as the natural elicitor (US), and, after the response to the paired stimuli has occurred, the previously neutral stimulus (CS) will now elicit that response (CR). If, for example, the sound of a bell (CS) is paired with the presentation of food (US), salivation (UR) can be elicited eventually by the bell alone (CR). It has been suggested that the UR and CR, although superficially similar, actually differ basically; for example, the chemical composition of saliva is different when it is naturally elicited than when it is conditioned to occur.

Classically conditioned responses have clearly defined properties, which distinguish them from operantly conditioned responses (Kimble, 1961). Such stimulus parameters of the CS as its intensity and duration are crucial, and the way in which the US and CS stimuli are paired, the interval between conditioning trials, and the regularity of the pairing also influence the CR. For example, short weak stimuli, which do not reliably occur together, constitute less than ideal conditions for classical conditioning. Even if strongly established, conditioned responses may quickly disappear (EXTINGUISH), once the stimulus contiguity is broken. When stimulus pairing is irregular, and conditioning accordingly weaker, extinction is even more rapid.

Operant conditioning, by contrast, is not concerned with modifying the eliciting conditions for behavior but with the processes by which the consequences of present behavior determine future behavior. If a response is followed by a pleasant or an unpleasant consequence, the probability of that response occurring again is changed. A pleasant consequence is called REINFORCEMENT and an unpleasant one PUNISHMENT. The former increases the probability of responding and the latter decreases it.

The basic concepts of operant conditioning were developed by the American school of behavior theory initiated by Thorndike. The original experiments were largely concerned with the learning of such complex tasks as mazes for rats or puzzle boxes for cats. The properties of operant conditioning, however, were most clearly defined by B. F. Skinner. In contrast to other theorists, who studied complex learned responses, Skinner believed that the principles of operant conditioning could be demonstrated most clearly when a simple response was studied. The lever press of a rat or the key peck of a pigeon served well for this purpose, and an automated apparatus for recording such behavior was developed, the so-called Skinner box. When placed in a small chamber with a lever on one wall, the rat emits a whole variety of responses, none of which is obviously elicited by stimuli in the environment. The lever is electrically connected so that when it is pressed a food reward drops into the cup below. Often the rat manipulates the lever by chance, and the process of reinforcement begins to operate. To speed this up, "free" reinforcements are given in the food well to encourage the rat to emit most of its behavior in the vicinity of the lever. Following "shaping" with reinforcement, further bar presses are likely to occur.

Operant and classical conditioning are clearly quite different procedures and so are their properties. One important difference between these two kinds of conditioning is the widely held belief that visceral responses controlled by the autonomic nervous system are always elicited rather than emitted and that emitted behavior is only controlled by the so-called voluntary motor nervous system. It therefore follows that classical conditioning involves mainly the autonomic nervous system and operant, the voluntary motor nervous system. This distinction has been widely accepted, and only in recent years has it been suggested that subtle and complex relationships may exist between these conditioning procedures. Whether they are controlled by the autonomic or by the voluntary motor nervous system, responses clearly do not occur in isolation. Behavior is a constantly changing profile of both kinds of responses, and it should not be surprising to find that both kinds are intermingled in conditioning.

Shapiro (1961) studied dogs that had been surgically prepared with chronic indwelling catheters in the duct of the parotid gland. In these dogs, a continuous record of salivary secretion was obtained while they were being reinforced with food for lever pressing. Reinforcement was given every 10 minutes, and the dogs salivated not only, as expected, after the food reinforcement, but also toward the end of the 10-minute fixed-interval period (Fig. 1-1). Furthermore, a high correlation between the magnitude of conditioned salivation and the number of lever presses during the fixed interval was observed. Clearly, this anticipatory salivation is closely tied to the operantly conditioned lever press, and it becomes meaningless to try to distinguish between elicited and emitted responses in a composite behavior of this kind. In considering whether hard and fast distinctions can be made between elicited and emitted responses, recent work from Miller's laboratory is relevant. This challenges

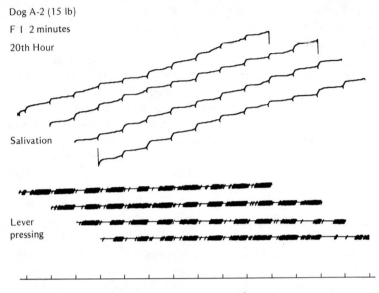

Dog A-2 (15 lb)

F I 2 minutes

20th Hour

Salivation

Lever
pressing

Time (2-minute intervals)

Fig. 1-1 Cumulative salivary responding and lever pressing by a dog, reinforced with food for lever presses on an F 12 schedule. *Upper:* cumulative salivary responses; *lower:* discrete lever presses. Reinforcements are
designated by the diagonal downstrokes of the cumulative pen. The salivary response clearly covaries with the schedule of food reinforcement.
(Reproduced from Shapiro, 1961.)

the dictum that elicited responses cannot be operantly conditioned. First, Miller and Carmona (1967) were able to show in
dogs that spontaneous increases or decreases in saliva output
could be maintained by appropriate reinforcement. The parotid
duct was canulated to allow measurement of saliva, the dogs
were made thirsty by water deprivation, and water was used as
the reinforcer. Such results, however, are inconclusive evidence
of autonomic instrumental conditioning. The skeletal muscles are
operative in the animal, and the observed visceral changes could

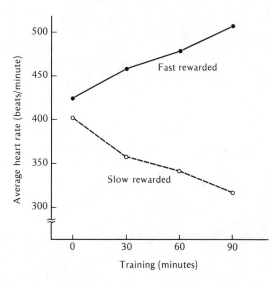

Fig. 1-2 Instrumental learning in groups rewarded for fast or slow heart rates. (Each point represents average beats per minute during 5 minutes). (Reproduced from Miller and DiCara, 1967.)

have been mediated via skeletal responses known to be instrumentally conditioned. To counter this criticism, Miller and DiCara (1967) subsequently prepared a curarized rat preparation in which all skeletal responses were eliminated. Spontaneous increases or decreases of heart rate were produced with electric stimulation at medial forebrain bundle sites known to show intracranial self stimulation in the rat (Fig. 1-2). In view of these findings, a potential value of operant autonomic conditioning for the treatment of psychosomatic illness has been proposed; patients might be trained to control their own aberrant heart rate or blood pressure, for example.

Despite the fact that elicited and emitted responses are so closely bound together in the fabric of normal behavior, classical conditioning procedures have hardly been used in the study of

9

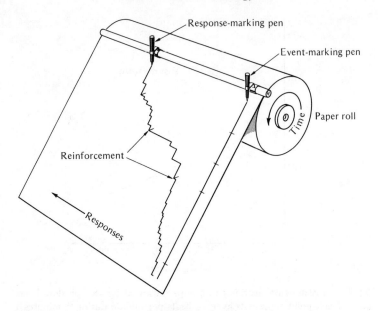

Fig. 1-3 A schematic drawing of the cumulative recorder. The paper un-rolls under the two pens with time. Each occurrence of the response moves the response-marking pen up one unit toward the top of the paper. Reinforcement is indicated by a hatch-mark on the cumulative record. Additional events during an experimental session can be indicated along the horizontal line at the bottom (or top) of the record by the event-marking pen. (Reproduced from Reynolds, 1968.)

the effects of drugs on behavior. Most of the rest of this chapter is, therefore, restricted to a consideration of the characteristics of operant conditioning.

The development of apparatus for automating reinforcement delivery and recording responses has played a large role in advancing experimental analyses of operant conditioning. Electromagnetic or solid-state switching circuits are used to control the stimuli in the testing chamber, the schedule of reinforcement, and the delivery of reinforcement when appropriate responses have been made. The responses to the lever, the key, or other device are counted, and their distribution over time plotted on cumulative recorders. This is a pen and paper recording method; the paper moves over a drum at a given speed, and each response moves the recording pen one step across the paper. The pen resets after crossing the paper. The rate and pattern of responding can immediately be seen: with high, regular rates of responding, the pen crosses the paper within a short time, whereas, with slow rates, the slope of the response line is proportionately less steep (Fig. 1-3).

Characteristics of reinforced behavior

Concepts of reinforcement

An event is identified as a reinforcer when it follows a response and there is a subsequent increase in the occurrence of that response or closely related ones. Reinforcement increases the probability of the recurrence of the immediately preceding behavior and may act as such either when it is presented (e.g., food) or when it is terminated (e.g., electric shock). The terms POSITIVE REINFORCEMENT for the presentation of pleasant events and NEGATIVE REINFORCEMENT for the removal of unpleasant events are commonly used. These terms are opposites, but since under both conditions the probability of responding increases, they can be misleading. It is perhaps better to simply talk of reinforcers and to describe the particular event. The concept of reinforcement is central to all behavior theory. Controversy centers rather on the nature of the responses that are strengthened and on the strengthening processes themselves. One school believes that animals learn relationships between external events and that reinforcement, although generally increasing the probability of learned behavior occurring, is not a prerequisite for the learned associations to be formed. By contrast, others view reinforcement as the means of forming learned associations. It is further contended that animals learned the *responses* made to external events rather than relationships between those events. The former theories are described as "cognitive" or "map in the head" and the latter "stimulus-response associative." Students are often asked, "do rats learn where to go or what to do." The behavior theories of Tolman and Hull polarize these controversies (Hilgard and Bower, 1966), but they are not our immediate concern. The demands of behavioral pharmacology are more consistent with Skinner's approach to behavior, which is basically a description of the variables influencing behavior in a particular situation, with no recourse to explanation. This is not to say that there are no underlying reasons for behavior, but simply that if behavior can be defined, described, and consistently manipulated, these reasons are irrelevant. Furthermore, as we shall see, explanations in terms of such internal variables as the motivation of fear or hunger can encourage parsimonious interpretations of behavior, which may be misleading. A rat presses a lever, obtains food, and subsequently presses the lever more frequently. To traditional behavior theorists, the animal is MOTIVATED to obtain food and learns the bar-pressing response because its INTERNAL DRIVE STATE is reduced by the food. To the Skinnerian, the probability of a bar-pressing response by a hungry animal increases if that response is followed by reinforcement.

Properties of reinforcers

The terms SATISFIER and ANNOYER from Thorndike's writings crystallize the nature of reinforcement. Certain events, innately or after experience, satisfy basic needs, and other events, by contrast, induce withdrawal. The tendency to withdraw from unpleasant events is innately strong and can be reliably induced in animals under experimental conditions. Species vary in what they find aversive; electric shock is effective in most species, but some species have particular aversions, which are useful experimentally, e.g., puffs of air to the cat. The need for satisfiers,

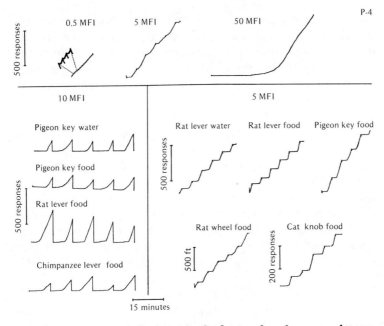

Fig. 1-4 Generality of characteristic fixed-interval performance, then acceleration to a maintained steady rate of responding. *Ordinate:* cumulative number of responses; *abscissa:* time. A fixed-interval schedule of presentation of food or water was in operation in all examples shown here. *Upper:* individual pigeon (P-4) pecking plastic key (food). Three different durations of the fixed interval (minute fixed interval, MFI) are shown; the general pattern persists despite the 100-fold change in the schedule parameter. Food presentations, ending each fixed interval, are marked by short diagonal strokes on the cumulative record. *Lower left:* performances under a 10-minute, fixed-interval schedule. Food or water presentations, ending each fixed interval, are marked by the resetting of the recording pen to the base line. *Lower right:* performances under a 5-minute, fixed-interval schedule. The species, the type of switch recording the response, and the reinforcements presented are indicated above the records. The pigeon pecks a plastic key with its beak; the rat and chimpanzee press a horizontal lever with their paws; the cat depresses a rounded knob with its paw. The rat turns the wheel by running; only a turn of 180° is reinforced, but the cumulative distance the wheel turns is recorded directly. (Reproduced from Kelleher and Morse, 1968.)

13

because of the general physiological characteristics of the animal, is variable, and DEPRIVATION is often used to ensure the potency of a satisfier for experimental purposes. The animal is deprived of a satisfier for a period of time, thus ensuring its reinforcing properties under experimental conditions. Food and water are most commonly used, but access to a receptive female for the male rat, salt, heat, electric stimulation of the brain, and infusion of such mood-changing drugs as amphetamine, cocaine, or morphine have all been used as reinforcing stimuli. For practical reasons, food deprivation and the use of food as a satisfier and electric shock as an annoyer dominate the experimental literature, and work is needed to demonstrate that the effects on behavior obtained by the presentation of food or withdrawal of shock are common to all reinforcers. It is impressive how similar response patterns are across species when a particular reinforcer is programmed to become available in the same way (Fig. 1-4).

Schedules of reinforcement

Regular reinforcement delivered quickly increases the probability of responding, but intermittent presentation of reinforcing stimuli reveals more clearly their ability to control behavior. Skinner and his collaborators in the 1930's and 1940's laid the groundwork for such studies by describing two basic manipulations or SCHEDULES of reinforcement, one determined by time and the other by frequency of responding.

The fixed-interval schedule (FI)

On this schedule, reinforcement becomes available at regular temporal intervals, e.g., every 5 minutes provided the animal makes an appropriate response. Irrespective of the animal's behavior during the interval, the first response that occurs after the 5 minutes have elapsed is reinforced. The animal could, therefore, make one response every 5 minutes and receive maximum reinforcement. After responding for a short period of time on such a schedule, animals do not do this, nor do they respond

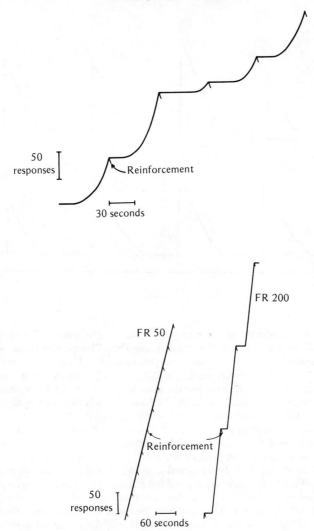

Fig. 1-5 *Upper:* Performance generated by a 1-minute, fixed-interval schedule; *lower:* performance generated by two different fixed-ratio (FR) schedules. (Reproduced from Reynolds, 1968.)

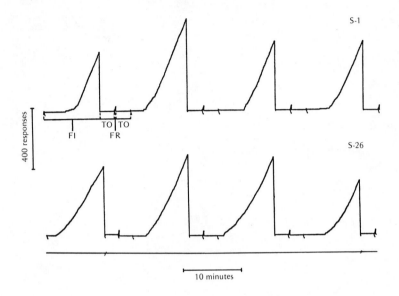

Fig. 1-6 Generality of characteristic multiple fixed-interval, fixed-ratio schedule performance in the squirrel monkey. The performances were maintained by food presentation (upper, monkey S-1) and by stimulus-shock termination (lower, monkey S-26). The sequence of visual stimuli and corresponding schedules was the same in the upper and lower records. At the beginning of the records, the FI 10-minute schedule was in effect in the presence of a white light. At the termination of the FI component, the recording pen reset to the base line. Following reinforcement, a pattern of horizontal lines was present for 2.5 minutes; during this time-out period (TO), responses had no programmed consequences. The next short diagonal stroke on the cumulative record indicates that the FR 30 component was in effect in the presence of a red light. Again the cumulative recording pen reset to the base line at reinforcement and was followed by the 2.5-minute TO component. This cycle was repeated throughout each session. At the bottom of the record for monkey S-26, the short diagonal strokes on the event line indicate electric shock presentations. The variation in the number of responses in fixed-interval components is normal. Note the similarities of the patterns of responding under these multiple FI FR food and shock schedules. (Reproduced from Kelleher and Morse, 1964.)

throughout the period. Their response pattern is said to be scalloped (Fig. 1-5). Immediately after a reinforcement, responding virtually ceases and then accelerates as the time for the next reinforcement approaches. The power of reinforcement in controlling behavior is illustrated by the fact that presentation of food *or* escape from an electric shock, when programmed on an FI, yields indistinguishable patterns of responding (Fig. 1-6). Such observations, incidently, undermine motivational explanations of behavior. It is difficult to explain, using the intervening variable of motivation, how food and fear can produce the same behavior. The explanation of the similarity of behavior lies not in the nature of the reinforcer but in the way it is programmed to occur.

Fixed-ratio schedules (FR)

By contrast, on ratio schedules, a fixed *number* of responses must be made before the reinforcement occurs, and thus, frequency of reinforcement is determined by frequency of response. Hence, FR schedules result in high regular response rates with only a short post-reinforcement pause (Fig. 1-5).

Both FI and FR schedules can be programmed to be variable.

The variable-interval schedule (VI)

Under these conditions, time again determines reinforcements, which occur at variable time intervals. A VI schedule has a range of inter-reinforcement delays around a mean value, which is used to designate the schedule (e.g., VI 1 minute has a mean inter-reinforcement time of 1 minute). This schedule generates a very high and sustained rate of responding due, it is said, to the uncertainty of the reinforcement.

The variable-ratio schedule (VR)

This schedule presents each reinforcement after a variable number of responses, and, again, there is a mean ratio-value used to designate the schedule. It generates a high regular rate of responding until the ratio demands become very large; then a waning of response, called straining, begins to appear as the animal has difficulty in meeting the response requirement.

Other reinforcement schedules

In addition to these commonly used schedules, a variety of modifications are used, constituting the subject matter of much operant conditioning research. The DRL (differential reinforcement of low rate of responding), for example, is now being used to greater extent in such applied research as behavioral pharmacology. The DRL is a *free-operant* schedule insofar as behavior is not parceled into discrete units by regular reinforcement. Reinforcement is programmed to occur after a certain period of time has elapsed since the previous response, but is actually given only when fewer than a specified number of responses has occurred during that period. If more than this number of responses has occurred, reinforcement is delayed until this low rate of responding has been achieved. The response requirement is stringent. A precise and steady rate within a narrow range of inter-response intervals is required, and a very high or a very low rate of responding reduces the reinforcement received. Such control is presumably behaviorally demanding, which probably explains why DRL performance takes a long time to stabilize and why it is so sensitive to physiological manipulation of the animal.

Equally precise high rates of responding are engendered by the differential reinforcement of high rates of responding (DRH), in which more than a certain number of responses are required during the inter-reinforcement time.

Avoidance of electric shock can also be programmed on a free operant schedule. Sidman gave his name to the procedure whereby a shock is programmed to occur regularly but is delayed by a fixed period every time a response is made. For example, shocks are given every 10 seconds until a response occurs; following a response, there is a 10-second delay until the next shock. Under such conditions, temporal discrimination develops and, as with DRL and DRH schedules, efficient behavior is achieved by responses occurring over a narrow range of inter-response intervals.

Multiple schedules

Multiple schedules are programmed by combining two or more schedules in a regular fashion. Alternation between two different schedules is most commonly used, for example, a multiple FI/FR schedule in which time and rate of responding alternate to determine reinforcement. A pattern of responding quickly develops, with the animal showing the characteristic scalloped pattern of responding during the FI component, followed by the high rate of responding during the FR component. Multiple schedules are of great value in studying drug effects, which are often partly determined by the ongoing rate of behavior. The stimulatory effect of amphetamine is one such example. It can be shown that the drug augments low rates of responding during the initial part of the FI components and depresses high rates during the FR components. To study a wider range of behavioral control, more than two components can be combined on a multiple schedule.

There are other interesting complex schedules that have not yet been much used in behavioral pharmacology. A compound schedule may reinforce a single response according to the requirement of *two or more* schedules of reinforcement simultaneously. CONJUNCTIVE FI/FR SCHEDULES are one such example; here a response is reinforced if a fixed interval of time has elapsed *and* if the fixed ratio of responses has been emitted. Another example are INTERLOCKING SCHEDULES; here a certain number of responses is required for reinforcement, but the absolute number varies with the time since the last reinforced response. The number may decrease or increase, and, under an increasing interlocking schedule, the demands of responding become so prohibitively large that reinforcement may never be obtained. Reynolds (1968) suggests that such a reinforcement principle operates in cumulative educational systems, where the requirements for success become increasingly large and where later success is precluded by an earlier lack of success. CONCURRENT SCHEDULES involve the reinforcement of two or more responses according to two or more simultaneous schedules. For example, pecking a red key may be reinforced on an FI, and pecking a separate blue key on an FR. Behavior is distributed between the keys in a complex manner, and a behavioral chain readily forms under these circumstances. If responding on one key happens to be reinforced when behavior is switched to that key, a chain of behavior is formed from the first key to the second key, which yields reinforcement. To prevent chaining, the schedule can be programmed so that behavior cannot be reinforced until a certain time after a switch, thus encouraging independent behavior under the two schedules.

In view of their relevance to most animal and human behavior, which is controlled by complex reinforcement contingencies rather than a single event, it is surprising that multiple schedules of this kind have not received more experimental investigation.

The most complex schedule so far discussed in this chapter involves no more than four simple schedules presented over a relatively short period of time. Experimental situations are now being explored in which the animal is controlled by programmed schedules for the whole day. Living environments are built in which dozens of different behaviors, their sequence, and their duration can be studied. The multi-operant repertoire represents an experimental effort to come to grips with this kind of complexity. Ferster (1966) has used a situation in which a pair of chimpanzees lived and worked in a semi-natural environment. They were free to work for food on certain cognitive problems, interact in a social environment, or sleep. Over a 5-year period, a remarkable orderly sequence of behavior was maintained with 4 to 6 hours of work and regular sleep. During the experiment, it proved necessary to replace the female animal, and this profoundly disrupted the behavioral stability of the male. Irrespective of responses to the new female, his work schedule was reduced, his appetite blunted. Experimental situations of this kind have an enormous potential for studying abnormal behavior and the ability of drugs to modulate such behavior. They offer the possibility of monitoring the whole output of behavior and the opportunity to manipulate experimentally the variables that control behavior.

Findley (1966) has pioneered such methods with humans, describing a situation in which the behavior of a 34-year-old male volunteer subject was studied over a 5-month period. This involved a chamber with eating, sleeping, and toilet facilities; a wide range of intellectual and physical activities could be enjoyed; and pleasant consequences of behavior, i.e. reinforcers like music and cigarettes were also offered. After 90 days, stress, which markedly influenced the distribution of behavior, was apparent—time spent on toilet facilities increased and intellectual activities decreased, while sleep occurred in more frequent, but shorter bouts. The potential of such methods for mimicking the total environment and for inducing abnormal behavior remains to be explored.

Discriminative stimuli

If responses are emitted and reinforced in the presence of a stimulus, that stimulus is called a DISCRIMINATIVE STIMULUS, or an S^D, and subsequently has information value for the animal by indicating the reinforcing contingency in operation. An S^D sets the occasion for emitted responses to occur. Stimuli that indicate that reinforcement is not operating are termed S^Δ. On a simple FI schedule, a house light may be the S^D; it is used to illuminate the testing chamber during the interval, but it is switched off immediately after the reinforcement, so that no light becomes the S^Δ. Light onset after the inter-trial interval signals the operation of the next FI. The specificity of discrimination control can be

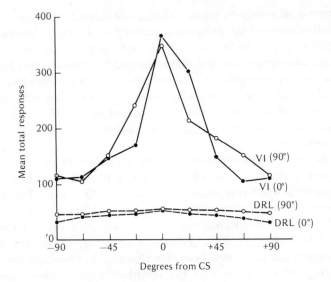

Fig. 1-7 Generalization gradients of tilt following training on a VI or a DRL schedule of reinforcement. Each group was composed of two subgroups, one trained with a vertical line as S^D (0°) and the other with a horizontal line as S^D (90°). The various stimuli presented during generalization testing are plotted on the abscissa in terms of the number of degrees they are from the S^D or CS (conditioned stimulus). (Reproduced from Hearst, Koresko, and Poppen, 1964.)

demonstrated in a stimulus generalization experiment. An animal responds in the presence of an S^D, e.g., a vertical line, and is subsequently exposed to a range of lines tilted from vertical to horizontal. The rate of responding to the generalization stimuli indicates the strength of the original discriminative control (Fig. 1-7). If the animal noticed the training stimulus, a large number of responses are emitted when this stimulus subsequently appears. Responding does not occur to unfamiliar stimuli. If, for some reason, the initial discrimination training is unsuccessful or if the animal has lost its discriminative capacity after training, stimuli presented during the generalization testing are responded to equally, and the gradient is said to be "flat." The generalization gradients produced in such experiments are "sharpened" if, during training, the animal is not reinforced for responding to a stimulus at one end of the range (the S^Δ), while being reinforced in the presence of the S^D, and if a reinforcement schedule that generates a high rate of responding is used during training.

Any sensory stimulus can theoretically acquire discriminative properties, although innate sensory capabilities and stimulus preferences determine the limits and priorities for stimulus control in any one species.

Conditioned reinforcers

If a stimulus that has no innate reinforcing property occurs with one that has, the neutral stimulus acquires reinforcing properties and becomes a CONDITIONED or SECONDARY REINFORCING STIMULUS. A classical example would be the noise of the food magazine delivery system in a Skinner box. Once responding is established with food and the accompanying noise, it can be maintained by presentation of the noise alone, in the absence of the food reinforcement. The behavior extinguishes less quickly than when there is no food and no noise. In addition to retarding extinction, conditioned reinforcers, like unconditioned ones, increase the probability of the recurrence of the responses that produce them. Conditioned reinforcers may be associated with the occurrence of pleasant reinforcers or with the avoidance of unpleasant ones.

Although it is theoretically possible to separate discriminative stimuli and conditioned reinforcers, it is difficult to do so in practice. If an S^D is present throughout the FI and the final reinforcing event, it can theoretically also acquire conditioned reinforcing properties. Natural behavior consists of sequences or chains of responses under stimulus control, and the conditioned reinforcers of one response may be the discriminative stimulus for the next, and so on along the chain. For example, a pigeon is presented with a blue key, an S^D. Pecking changes the color to red (CR); the key color change is a conditioned reinforcer for the response that produced it, and then the sustained color becomes the S^D for the next emitted response, a pedal press that changes the key color again. This chain of S^D and CR stimuli continues until a final response results in reinforcement. Key color change here is a conditioned reinforcer because, in the final segment of the chain, it is associated with food reinforcement. The conditioned reinforcing strength of a stimulus is in proportion to its distance from the unconditioned reinforcer, and the length of functional chains is limited for this reason.

There is considerable theoretical controversy about the mechanism of conditioned reinforcement that can be usefully investigated with chaining procedures. Traditionally, conditioned reinforcers were studied by pairing the potential conditioned reinforcers with an unconditioned reinforcing stimulus such as food and then assessing the ability of the conditioned reinforcer to maintain behavior in the absence of food. The behavior, thus, gradually extinguishes as the experiment progresses. If, however, conditioned reinforcers are set up in chains, those not directly associated with the terminal food reinforcement maintain behavior in the early parts of the chain. Their properties and ability to maintain behavior can thus be assessed on a maintained behavioral base line without extinction procedures being introduced.

Several competing theories have been proposed to explain how conditioned reinforcers come to control behavior. The most satisfactory explanation at present seems to be that the neutral stimulus becomes a reinforcing stimulus by classical conditioning between the unconditioned reinforcing stimulus and the neutral stimulus.

Extinction

If a strongly maintained behavior is suddenly no longer reinforced, extinction follows and the behavior gradually wanes. The characteristics of extinction depend on the schedule of rein-

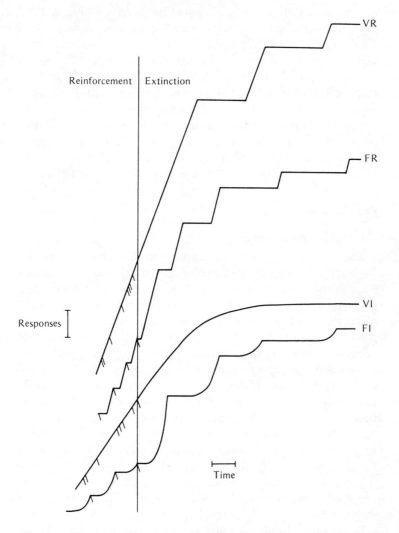

Fig. 1-8 The general course and features of extinction following reinforcement on each of four simple schedules, VR, FR, VI, FI. (Reproduced from Reynolds, 1968.)

forcement that originally maintained the behavior (Fig. 1-8). If every response had been reinforced (continuous reinforcement, CRF), then extinction is rapid. By contrast, if reinforcement has been irregular and generated a high rate of responding, as for example on a VR, extinction takes much longer, and bursts of responding are seen in the absence of reinforcement. It has been suggested that the rate of extinction depends on the ease with which the animal can discriminate the change in the reinforcement contingency. After CRF, extinction is immediately apparent, but, if reinforcement has been irregular, the change to extinction is much more difficult to discriminate.

Punishment

Concepts of punishment

The effects of aversive stimuli on behavior challenge behavior theory. As we have seen earlier, escape from or avoidance of such aversive stimuli as electric shock can act as a *reinforcing event* to increase the probability of the behavior that brought about the relief from shock. On the other hand, aversive stimuli presented under conditions where escape or avoidance are not possible clearly suppress ongoing behavior. First, it had to be established how escape from or avoidance of aversive stimuli could be fitted into reinforcement theory and, second, if punishment were a special case of reinforcement or an entirely independent means of manipulating behavior. Theorists have, in turn, either ignored these problems or have made them central to general theories of behavior. Many workers have focused on the aversive stimulus as being central to any theory of punishment and have considered the ways in which aversive stimuli can modify behavior. Given the procedure in operation, animals may, on the one hand, escape from or avoid shock, and, on the other hand, their behavior may be suppressed by shock. Observers of natural behavior might well characterize such defensive behaviors as flight and immobility. Theoretically speaking, flight is maintained by shock acting as a negative reinforcer. A negative reinforcer, like a positive reinforcer, increases the probability of responding (in this case, flight from the aversive stimulus). In contrast, responding may be suppressed by the presentation of shock, which is then considered to be a punisher. Despite the opposite influences on response probability of reinforcement and punishment, there have been continuing efforts to find a unitary explanation for the widely varying effects of aversive stimuli on behavior.

If we could convince ourselves that reinforcement was operating in all the procedures, we might be able to accommodate all the results of aversive stimuli into reinforcement theory. This was Skinner's attitude to punishment. He saw it as a special case of reinforcement, where avoidance of shock was mediated not by the observed reduction in responding, but by an increase in the probability of an internal and unobservable response in the animal. Thus, with punishment, as with reinforcement, a response probability (i.e., the response being not to respond) increases. This explanation is attractively parsimonious, but recourse to unobservable events for explanatory purposes does not produce an easily testable hypothesis. It would be convenient to encompass all the effects of aversive stimuli within reinforcement theory, but there is a strong current of opinion that maintains that a decrease in response probability to aversive stimuli (punishment) is a different process, which can be procedurally distinguished from the other varied effects of shock. There is also evidence that different neural systems underlie active and passive defensive reactions (McCleary, 1966) and that they are differentially affected by a variety of drugs (Kelleher and Morse, 1964). Thus punishment should be considered an independent behavioral contingency. It, therefore, seems inappropriate, as some recent workers have done, to lump together aversive stimuli used as reinforcers and discriminative stimuli used as punishers. In theoretical ferment of this kind, the existence of a confusing terminology is almost inevitable. We do not feel that

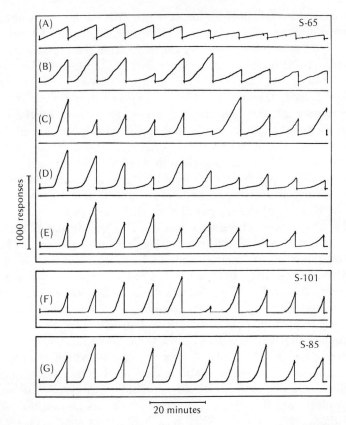

Fig. 1-9 Patterns of responding under different experimental conditions. *Ordinate:* cumulative number of responses per 10-minute fixed interval; *abscissa:* time. The recording pen was reset to the base line at the termination of each fixed interval. (A) Schedule of shock-postponement and 10-minute fixed-interval (FI 10) schedule of shock-presentation programmed concurrently (10th session after introduction of FI 10, monkey S-65). (B) FI 10 shock-presentation only (21st session after elimination of shock-postponement schedule, monkey S-65). (C) FI 10 shock-presentation, 30-second time-out period after each shock (14th session after introduction of time-out, monkey S-65). (D) FI 10 shock-presentation, no time-out (16th session after removal of time-out, monkey S-65). (E) FI 10 shock-

28

it is necessary to consider the controversy in detail here, and punishment will be considered only in procedural terms.

Electric shocks may increase or decrease responding, but it is the procedure, not the stimulus, that is central to the matter of punishment and reinforcement. This has been dramatically demonstrated by McKearney (1968a). Squirrel monkeys were trained on a shock postponement schedule, with every press of a lever delaying the shock for 30 seconds; this schedule elicited a steady rate of responding. An FI 10-minute shock presentation was then programmed concurrently (Fig. 1-9A). The shock postponement was eliminated, and the only consequence of responding was an intense shock every 10 minutes. Under these conditions, a "scalloped" pattern of responding quickly emerged, which was indistinguishable from patterns controlled by food presentation every 10 minutes (Fig. 1-9). This particular training history resulted in monkeys responding to receive an intense shock that, under other conditions, would eliminate behavior. The shock was controlling behavior as a reinforcer.

Properties of punishment

A procedure described by Geller (1962) illustrates most directly the suppressive effects of punishment. A rat is trained to press a lever for food on a VI schedule. After high rates of lever pressing are induced, shock is introduced. The rat is shocked through the feet each time a response is made to the lever, and,

---

presentation, 30-second time-out reinstated (fourth session after reinstatement of time-out, 63rd session after elimination of shock-postponement schedule, monkey S-65). (F) Stabilized performance of monkey S-101 under the FI 10 schedule of shock-presentation with a 30-second time-out after shock (57th session after elimination of shock-postponement schedule). (G) Stabilized performance of monkey S-85 under the FI 10 schedule of shock-presentation with a 30-second time-out after shock (67th session after elimination of shock-postponement schedule). The variation in numbers of responses in successive intervals within a session is typical of fixed-interval schedules in general. (Reproduced from McKearney, 1968.)

although responses are still reinforced on the VI as well as punished, the over-all rate of responding is severely depressed.

This procedure has been used very successfully in behavioral pharmacology to characterize drugs that counter the suppressive effects of aversive stimuli. For example, minor tranquilizers, such as the benzodiazepines, dramatically reinstate behavior suppressed by electric shock, and the use of this technique by Geller et al. (1962) provides the most specific test for this important group of drugs. Punishment programmed in this way is called IM-MEDIATE punishment to denote the fact that it follows a response on a regular time relationship and to distinguish it from ADVENTI-TIOUS punishment, which occurs irrespective of the animal's responses. A rat, for example, could be shocked halfway through a VI period irrespective of whether the lever had just been pressed. The interval between response and shock would then be highly variable.

The difference between adventitious and immediate punishment would seem to be of considerable behavioral significance. One might suppose that punishment of known origin would be reacted to in a different way from punishment that apparently occurs randomly. But, in fact, since the distinction between the

---

Fig. 1-10 (A) Effect of food deprivation during fixed-ratio punishment of food-reinforcement responses. Every 100th response is being punished (160 V) at the moment indicated by the short oblique lines on the response curves. The food reinforcements (not shown) are being delivered according to a 3-minute variable schedule. (B) Stable performance during fixed-ratio punishment at several fixed-ratio values from FR 1 to FR 1000. The oblique lines on the response curve indicate the delivery of a punishment (240 V). The food reinforcements (not indicated) are being delivered according to a 3-minute variable interval schedule. (C) Effect of punishment intensity during fixed-ratio punishment. Every 50th response is being punished at the moment indicated by the oblique lines on the response curves. Each response curve represents the performance during the first 60 minutes of different sessions. The food reinforcements (not indicated) are being delivered according to a 1-minute variable interval. (Reproduced from Azrin et al., 1963.)

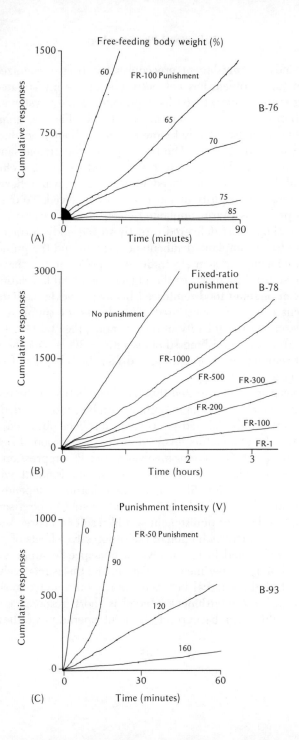

two kinds of punishment procedures has been recognized, this fascinating problem has not been adequately investigated.

Azrin and Holtz (1966) have provided a most systematic description of immediate punishment. To be effective, immediate punishment must reliably follow responses. Foot shock has been found to be unreliable. The resistance of the animal, and particularly of the skin of the feet, varies and so does the effectiveness of the shock. The speed of leg withdrawal reflexes also determines the severity of shock actually received. To overcome these problems, Azrin implanted electrodes in various animals, so that shock was delivered directly to the body surface. Gold electrodes are implanted subcutaneously around the pubic bone of the pigeon, and skin electrodes are applied to the shaved tail of the squirrel monkey. In the pigeon, predictable relationships between ongoing food-reinforced behavior and immediate punishment can be demonstrated. The degree of suppression depends on (a) the severity of deprivation (Fig. 1-10A), (b) the strength of the punishing stimulus (Fig. 1-10C), (c) the schedule of reinforcement operating, and (d) the schedule of punishment (Fig. 1-10B).

It has been demonstrated that the delay between the response and the punishment is an important variable, and a graded effect with increasingly delayed punishment has been observed. There appear to be two factors involved in the suppression of behavior by punishment. One factor involves a specific suppression of the punished response by the association of punishment with the emission of behavior. Since associative learning depends upon the temporal relationship between the events to be associated, increasing delay of punishment would result in poorer learning, with a consequent reduction of the suppressive effects of punishment. The second factor involves a non-specific suppression of behavior in the experimental situation, and this is relatively independent of the interval between the response and punishment. If the response-punishment interval is short, response suppression should occur because of the joint operation of these two factors. If punishment is delayed beyond the limits within which associative learning can occur, however, any suppression induced by punishment must be due solely to the non-specific effects of shock in the situation, and further increases in delay of punishment will have no further effect. A study of the suppression of worm eating in goldfish with electric shock gives such results (Myer and Ricci, 1968). Goldfish were placed in bowls for daily feeding sessions during which 20 small clusters of Tubifex worms were presented at 150-second intervals. When the fish were reliably taking worms during the feeding sessions, shock was administered through electrodes immersed in the water on two sides of the bowls either when a fish seized a cluster of worms or 2.5, 5, 10, or 20 seconds *after* the feeding response. At any particular delay, a suppression threshold was determined by increasing the intensity of the shock by 5 V each day until a criterion of 15 failures or more to feed on 3 successive days was reached. The amount of punishment required to suppress feeding was an increasing function of delay of punishment. The delay of punishment gradient increased sharply as the delay of punishment increased from 0 to 10 seconds. Further increase in the response-shock interval had no effect on the suppression threshold. It is suggested that at very low intensities punishment was suppressive only if it were closely associated with the emission of the response. At longer delays (up to 10 seconds) increased intensity of shock was required to suppress feeding. Increasing the delay from 10 to 20 seconds presumably had no additional effect because the suppression exhibited was due entirely to the generalized suppressive effects of shock in the experimental situation, rather than to more explicit associative learning.

It is interesting that certain aversive stimuli do not appear to show such a gradient. Some rat poisons produce unpleasant effects in the animal long after ingestion, and yet the rats develop "bait shyness." This question has received experimental attention and Revusky (1968) finds that if rats are irradiated to induce radiation sickness 7 hours after drinking sucrose, the subsequent consumption of this solution is greatly reduced. Furthermore, aversion to food that has caused illness is associated with the taste and odor of that food and not its appearance. Garcia and Koelling (1966) report experiments in which rats drank lithium chloride (which causes a gastrointestinal disturbance) in the presence of a discriminative stimulus, a light-click stimulus. When subsequently offered, in the presence of the same discriminative stimulus, salt solution (which tastes like the lithium solution) and water, the salt solution was rejected and the water drunk, despite the fact that the visual and auditory discriminative stimulus associated with the lithium was presented during the test trials.

Punishing stimuli, like reinforcers, may act simultaneously as discriminative stimuli. This property of punishing stimuli interacts with their response-suppressing action and is the source of much of the confusion that surrounds punishment theory. Punishment may signal further punishing or reinforcing events. Dinsmoor (1952) randomly alternated fixed periods of time during which punishment was programmed, with periods of no shock. The rats quickly learned that a punished response meant further punishment, and the probability of responding dropped; in contrast, two unpunished responses meant no punishment, and response rates rapidly increased. In a pigeon experiment (Azrin et al., 1963), FR punishment was programmed. At first there was complete suppression, but, gradually, the pigeons learned that responses were never punished immediately after a shock, and responding reappeared at the start of each FR. Punishment may also signal reinforcement and can lead to increased rates of responding. Holtz and Azrin (1961) alternated periods of intermittent food reinforcement with periods of extinction, and all responses were punished during the periods of reinforcement. Here, again, the occurrence of the punishing stimulus is used to detect reinforcement; this reveals a paradoxical effect of punishment—

the rate of responding was higher in the presence of punishment than in the absence of punishment.

This effect of punishment is comparable to the use of a neutral stimulus, such as the click of a food magazine associated with food reinforcement. The click becomes a conditioned reinforcer, increasing rates of responding during extinction. In the Holtz and Azrin experiment (1961), a punishing stimulus is substituted for a neutral one, but procedurally speaking it is, nevertheless, a conditioned reinforcer. As with reinforcement, associated stimuli may be discriminative, they may act as conditioned reinforcers, or both; it is equally difficult to dissociate these properties of stimuli that become associated with punishment. To complete the correspondence of the two processes, as with conditioned reinforcement, conditioned punishment is being studied with chaining procedures. Furthermore, it is thought that neutral stimuli acquire their information value with regard to punishment by a classical conditioning process. On the Estes-Skinner (1941) procedure (see p. 38), the warning signal (CS) is paired with the shock (US) until the unconditioned response of anxiety or fear (UR) is elicited by the CS.

ABNORMAL BEHAVIOR

Introduction

Behavior is under the constant control of a wide range of internal and external stimuli. When the animal no longer responds to these controlling stimuli in the usual way, we talk about maladaptive or abnormal behavior. In addition to its inherent scientific interest, behavioral science is of practical value when it increases our understanding of the conditions that disrupt behavioral control and of the nature of the abnormal behavior. Unfortunately, the complex nature of normal control makes it difficult to isolate and identify a particular contingency that is disrupting behavior. Furthermore, there is a very fine and ambiguous line between normal and abnormal behavior, and often a behavior described as abnormal in one context is perfectly normal in another. Aggression is one such example. Aggression includes threat and attack and can be seen when an animal kills its prey, for example, rat killing in the cat. It is also seen when animals fight over territory, but it can be equally well induced in a pigeon if reinforcement is suddenly terminated in an operant conditioning situation; is this aggression normal or abnormal?

It is essential to understand the control of normal behavior before turning to the abnormal, and yet it is toward the abnormal that behavioral pharmacology should be turning, since much of its concern centers on drugs that are used to modify or induce abnormal behavioral responses in man.

There is every reason to think that man's behavior is controlled by the same basic contingencies as is behavior in the pigeon. The difference in man is that his interaction with the environment is far more complex, and the mosaic of controlling factors is accordingly much larger and more difficult to identify. But progress can be made in understanding complex human behavior even by applying the comparatively simple principles gleaned from the pigeons' behavior. Ferster (1966) draws analogies of this kind and says, "Animal experiments do not tell us why a man acts but they do tell us where to look for factors of which his behavior is a function." He refers to the Estes-Skinner procedure where behavior is suppressed when an animal comes to anticipate a punishing stimuli after a warning signal; and Ferster draws an analogy with the lack of behavior or abnormal behavior often seen in a dentist's waiting room or subjectively experienced when one is waiting to consult a doctor about worrisome symptoms—a magazine scanned and not read, conversation muted. Ferster maintains that when drugs are used to ameliorate mental illness, they do not induce normality by creating behavior missing from the repertoire. Drugs can only influence the existing repertoire, modulating the complex relationship between controlling stimuli and behavioral responses.

Model systems for studying abnormal behavior

As we have seen, punishment provides the complementary force to reinforcement and, together, these events largely determine behavioral output at any one time. If we speak anthropomorphically, behavior is considered to be motivated on the one hand by the seeking and expectancy of pleasing events and on the other by the avoiding (or withdrawing from) and fear of unpleasant ones. It could be claimed that the emotional state of the organism reflects at any one time the balance of these motivating forces. The elation after reinforcement or the depression of behavior consequent to punishment should not be considered abnormal, but, clearly, the response to such events can become abnormally accentuated and markedly disrupt ongoing behavior.

In discussing normal behavioral control, we have tried to stress the fact that the way reinforcing and punishing events are scheduled is more important for our understanding of behavior than the nature of the events themselves. The same is true for behavior that appears to be abnormal. If such behavior is analyzed in sufficient detail, it is often possible to see that disordered behavior can be explained and that it has evolved from a particular combination and sequence of perfectly normal events (Sidman, 1960).

The development of model systems for studying abnormal behavior has, to a great extent, involved the manipulation of unpleasant events and the use of shock as a stimulus to induce marked changes in the motivational and emotional state of animals. Such powerful negative reinforcers as loud noise, however, have been identified and may prove to be more relevant to human behavior.

With regard to mental illness and abnormal behavior in man,

there is a tendency to think that studies of social behavior, development, and maternal deprivation in animals are more relevant than the operant conditioning of simple responses. This may be so, but, until we have identified more fully the spectrum of controlling stimuli for these aspects of complex behavior, they do not provide useful experimental base lines. It remains a fact that, at present, some of the simple techniques for manipulating behavior with aversive stimuli are the most useful for illustrating how, under certain conditions, stimuli may induce abnormal behavior and how drugs can modify this relationship.

The use of electric shock to induce emotional behavior

Introduction

Shock can be used to sustain or suppress behavior. Its sustaining function on escape and avoidance schedules produces, as a corollary, facets of emotional behavior that have long been considered models of abnormal behavior. Since these procedures have been extensively discussed in the literature (Kimble, 1961), attention here will be given to punishment schedules as inducers of abnormal behavior.

A punisher is a stimulus that can suppress behavior preceding its presentation. The punishing stimulus, as discussed earlier, may either occur irrespective of the responses (adventitious or noncontingent) or it can be initiated by the animals' responses (immediate or contingent or response produced). The work on immediate punishment was described earlier in the chapter.

Adventitious shock

Several procedures involving adventitious punishment have been of continuing interest with respect to abnormal behavior. The general principle is to superimpose shocks on behavior maintained by some other motivation or state. A modification of this principle, devised originally by Estes and Skinner (1941),

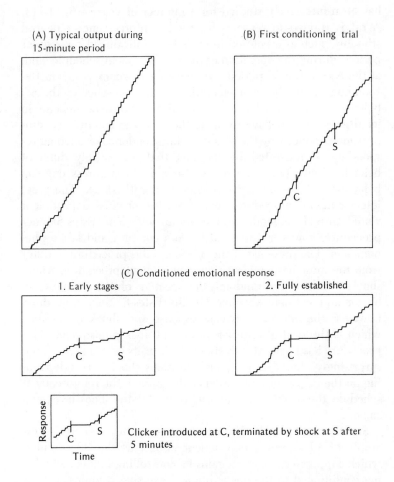

(A) Typical output during 15-minute period

(B) First conditioning trial

(C) Conditioned emotional response

1. Early stages 2. Fully established

Response

Time

Clicker introduced at C, terminated by shock at S after 5 minutes

Fig. 1-11 The conditioning of suppression during presentation of a pre-aversive stimulus. Typical VI performance reinforced by food is presented in (A). (B) shows the effect of a brief shock (S) on this VI performance. (C₁) and (C₂) illustrate early and late conditioned suppression with progressively fewer responses emitted during the clicks. (Reproduced from Hunt and Brady, 1951.)

has been intensively studied for a number of years (Fig. 1-11). A rat is trained to respond for food reinforcement. A neutral stimulus, such as a colored light, is then introduced for regular periods during the operation of the reinforcement schedule, and, at the end of the S^D period, an unavoidable shock is given. Responding gradually changes so that, in the presence of the S^D, behavior is suppressed, and reinforced responding occurs only in its absence. The behavior during the S^D is the conditioned suppression produced by the shock. Its independence of ongoing responding is illustrated by the fact that, in entirely different behavioral situations, the S^D is also able to suppress ongoing behavior that has never been associated with shock. The great interest in this procedure stems from the original hope that it would provide a model system of anxiety. The Estes-Skinner procedure, however, turns out to be a complex and labile phenomenon. The presence of the S^D causes this procedure to differ from the most basic adventitious punishment procedure, where shocks would occur randomly irrespective of the animal's behavior and without warning. On the Estes-Skinner procedure, however, the interval between response and shock is variable, which is the central criterion of adventitious punishment. This procedure has been extensively studied for its own sake, and, not surprisingly, the effect of the adventitious shock varies depending on the degree of motivation of the animal, the reinforcement schedule, the quality and intensity of the S^D, the shock level, and so on.

Strictly speaking, the Estes-Skinner procedure is a special example of adventitious punishment insofar as the S^D stimulus, which suppresses behavior, gains its controlling influence by being conditioned to the unconditioned aversive stimulus. Unpredictable shocks that occur without the presence of any overt discriminative cues will also produce marked changes in ongoing behavior. In natural situations, the source of aversive stimulation is often another organism, and the reaction is to engage in various species—typical aggressive and defensive behaviors. Azrin and his colleagues have recently studied such elicited aggression under laboratory conditions. Confined rats when shocked, fight vigorously (O'Kelly and Steckle, 1939). The fighting behavior differs in wild and domesticated breeds of the same animal. If wild rats are used, the fighting involves attack. Ulrich, Hutchinson, and Azrin (1965) report, however, that, in laboratory-bred rats, the response is a form of "defensive" fighting, or boxing, and it may be that domestication has somewhat modified aggressive responses in such situations from attack to defensive behavior. Elicited aggression is influenced by the stimulus conditions under which it occurs. Rats paired with hamsters modify their boxing posture to suit the size of their adversary, or, when shocked in the presence of various inanimate objects, they attack some objects preferentially. Squirrel monkeys attack, by biting, any animate or inanimate object when their tails are shocked, but, again, stimuli vary in their ability to elicit biting. Given the choice of a rubber ball or metal box, the monkeys invariably attack the former. Biting after shock can be shown to be rewarding in that monkeys will learn to pull a chain to gain access to a rubber bite ball when shocked (Azrin et al., 1965). In several species, the intensity and frequency of biting attack varies with the intensity and duration of the shock (Hutchinson et al., 1968). Other aversive stimuli such as a heated floor with the rat and tail pinching with the monkey have been shown to elicit aggression.

The work on shock-elicited aggression has encouraged the view that there is some fundamental and unique relationship between pain and aggression. It is more likely, however, that moderate pain potentiates any active behavior that has a high probability of occurring. Rats in crowded living conditions show aggressive-defensive behavior, and, if shock is added to the situation, these behaviors are even more likely to be released. Support for this interpretation comes from observations that other forms of behavior are potentiated by adventitious shock. Male rats were placed with receptive females and the frequency of copulation noted during several exposures (Barfield and Sachs, 1968). The males were then shocked in the presence of the females, and it was found that copulation occurred more often. Immediately after each shock, the female was paired and mounted, and the post-ejaculatory refractory period, when copulation does not occur, significantly decreased. A non-social behavior that has been studied in this way is eating. Ullman (1951) deprived rats of food and then studied their food intake during twenty 1-minute sessions. During the first 5 seconds of every minute, shock was administered, and, after several test days, it was observed that the greatest amount of eating occurred *during* these shock periods and the least in the 5 seconds *after* the shock.

A comparison of immediate and adventitious punishment in suppressing and disrupting behavior

As we have seen, adventitious punishment may, if given in certain situations, actually promote species specific behaviors that are actually occurring or that may relate to the particular situation. More commonly, if administered at certain intensity levels, and in situations where such relevant species specific behavior as fighting or mating are not occurring, adventitious punishment will produce responses incompatible with ongoing behavior. Shock does not have to be conditioned to a discriminative stimulus as in the Estes-Skinner procedure. Immediate punishment is more straightforward and effectively suppresses both operant and respondent behavior under all conditions. Solomon (1964) has suggested that consummatory responses are more readily suppressed by punishment than instrumental acts.

Some attempts have been made to compare the suppressive effects of the two shock procedures. Hunt and Brady (1955) trained rats to respond for food on a 1-minute VI schedule during 12-minute daily sessions; conditioning sessions were then introduced, and from the 4th to the 6th minute of the session a clicking sound was present. Some rats were shocked when they responded (immediate) during this period, and others received inescapable shocks (Estes-Skinner adventitious) at the end of the period. Lever pressing in the presence of the clicking sound was equally suppressed in both groups, but closer inspection of the over-all behavior revealed interesting differences.

1. The adventitious group showed greater suppression when the conditioned stimulus was not present.

2. When, at the end of the experiment, sessions were given with the conditioned stimulus but no shock, responding in the immediate punishment group recovered more quickly than in the adventitious group.

3. During shock-induced suppression, the behaviors observed in the two groups differed; the adventitious animals displayed crouching and immobility, whereas the response contingent group were more active and frequently made anticipatory responses to the lever. In the latter case, the suppressive effect of punishment seemed to be very closely tied to the lever-pressing response.

Azrin (1956) trained pigeons to peck a key for food on a 3-minute variable-interval schedule. After responding was well established, the response key was alternately illuminated with an orange and a blue light every 2 minutes. The food reinforcement schedule remained in effect regardless of the color of the key, but a shock contingency was introduced in the presence of the orange light. Each animal was subjected to four different shock procedures, but shock-free recovery periods were interposed between the different procedures. Under the adventitious shock conditions, an inescapable shock was administered either a fixed or a variable time after the orange light came on. Thus, the orange light was a warning signal for an impending shock, regardless of the animals' behavior. Under the punishment conditions, a shock was "due" some fixed or variable time after onset of the orange light but was not administered unless the pigeons pecked the key. If no response occurred between the time the punishment contingency came into effect and the end of the 2-minute stimulus period, the color of the key was changed, and no shock was administered. There were variations in the pattern of responding in the presence of the orange light depending upon whether the shock occurred after a fixed or variable interval, but, with either schedule of administration of shock, there was much greater suppression of responding under the response contingent procedure than when shock conditions were independent of behavior.

Immediate punishment, unlike adventitious shock, will also suppress instinctive or consummatory behaviors. Mouse killing by certain strains of rats was studied by Myer (1966, 1968). Immediate punishment of the mouse-seizing responses dramatically suppressed the killing behavior, whereas similar adventitious punishment when the mouse was presented but had not been attacked did not suppress killing. These findings suggest that the suppression of attack behavior does not depend upon the association of shock with the stimulus that arouses attack, but rather on the association of shock with the attacking. Similar results have been obtained with dogs who were shocked either when food was presented or as eating started.

Brady (1958) extended his investigation of shock procedures to study the somatic consequences of adventitious punishment, using intensive work schedules involving avoidance responding to eliminate shocks to produce a high incidence of such gastrointestinal lesions as ulcers. In his well-known "executive monkey" study, monkeys were yoked together so that they received an identical series of shocks, but one of the pair initiated the shocks by his responses, while the other passively received them at unpredictable times. The "responsible" animals, rather than the yoked controls, developed the lesions. The length of the work session was an important variable in these experiments; 6-hour avoidance–6-hour rest regimes produced ulcers, whereas alternated 30-minute sessions were better tolerated. These results must be treated with caution, however, since the monkeys were not assigned to groups in a balanced order. The animals who learned the conditioned response first in this experiment became the "responsible" subjects. A more recent study of Weiss et al. (1968) did not suffer from this defect and showed that, in the rat, the yoked subjects receiving adventitious shock lost weight, developed larger stomach ulcers more frequently, defecated more frequently, and showed a greater inhibition of drinking in the shock situation than rats who were able to avoid shock by their own actions.

Although there seems to be general agreement that conditioned responding is suppressed to a greater extent by immediate than by adventitious punishment, the picture is not so clear when unconditioned responses are monitored under these two conditions. More physiological and behavioral research is needed in this area, for we might suppose that the differences between self-initiated and adventitious punishment would be of great relevance to our understanding of the effects of aversive stimuli on human behavior.

Studies of aversive stimuli other than electric shock

Introduction

The preoccupation with shock as an aversive stimulus has had unfortunate theoretical implications. In his theory of avoidance behavior, Mowrer (1939) proposed that aversive stimuli induce fear, which is motivating, and that fear is always a conditioned response based on the association of some previously non-aversive stimulus with pain. There are, however, good grounds for questioning the assumption that all fears are conditioned responses of this kind. Many stimuli that are not painful or do not lead to painful consequences can be used as negative reinforcers or punishers and are highly aversive if their behavioral effects are observed. The termination of noise, for example, has been shown to reinforce escape behavior in humans (Azrin, 1958), monkeys (Klugh and Patton, 1959), cats, rats, and mice. Response-contingent noise suppresses responding in a similar range of species. Intense light will motivate escape learning and can serve as an unconditioned stimulus for avoidance learning. Forced swimming in cold water is highly aversive to rats (Glaser, 1910). Being touched by a hot or cold metal plate and blasted with air evoke active escape. Complex patterns of auditory and visual stimuli are apparently aversive in that they release typical patterns of defensive behavior in various species; ducklings, for example, freeze at the sight of a hawk. Bronson (1968) has reviewed studies of the ontogenetic development of certain of these species-specific reactions to fear-arousing stimuli—particularly novel stimuli—and suggests how this kind of fear can disrupt behavior after normal development has been disrupted by isolation or maternal deprivation.

Novelty as an aversive stimulus

Bronson (1968) suggests that reactions to such non-visual aversive stimuli as pain and loud noises should be called "distress reactions" and that these can be observed at a very early stage of development. He distinguishes between these distress reactions and the fear of novelty, i.e., unfamiliar visual stimuli, which develops later. A fair degree of stimulation at this stage of development appears to be a prerequisite for the maturation of normal responses to novelty. Levine's studies (1962) show that rats given excitatory stimulation associated with handling or electric shock are subsequently less fearful of novel situations than rats not given this experience. These kinds of experiments suggest that deprivation during development can markedly change responses to aversive stimuli. It could well be that partial deprivation occurs even when the mother is present, due perhaps to unusual characteristics of the infant or the mother. In either case, some early human psychopathology may have roots in disturbances beginning in the initial postnatal period.

Encoding the familiar is a prerequisite to the fear of novelty. Human infants must be capable of visual memory before a fear of visual novelty can develop. This seems to develop at about 2 months of age. Fantz (1964) found that before 2 months infants showed no difference in their reactions to new versus previously presented visual patterns, whereas after 2 months they spent less time gazing at "familiar" than at novel patterns. By 3 months, infants begin to smile less at strangers and from 6 months show attachment to a specific "mothering" person. Although physical contact seems to be paramount in allaying distress reactions, the mere presence of the mother within the child's visual field will allay tensions provoked by novel situations. It seems that infants begin to be disturbed by visual novelty at the time comfort is found in a visual awareness of the mother's presence. In monkeys, the fear of novelty and mother attachment occur at about 3 weeks of age (Harlow and Harlow, 1965). In the human, there is a gradual development of the ability to deal with novel visual experiences in the absence of the mother.

In view of such developmental evidence, it is not surprising to find that deprivation can permanently disturb the reaction to novelty. At the Yerkes laboratories, chimpanzees were separated from their mother at birth, and Davenport and Menzel (1963) report that at 2 years of age such animals reacted by crouching, rocking, and swaying when presented with novel objects in their home cage. They made no attempt to withdraw from the objects, and the stereotyped behavior continued for several hours. The chimps seemed intensely fearful and did not approach and explore the objects. These mother-separated animals had been observed throughout the 2-year period, and it was clear that stereotyped behavior occurred even in the familiar environment of the home cage but was further intensified by novelty. Rhythmic rocking, swaying, or turning movements were seen as well as such repetitive activities as thumb-sucking and exaggerated chewing movements. Monkeys reared without a mother show similar behavior patterns. Comparable observations have been made in institution-reared infants (Bridges, 1932), and stereotyped rocking is characteristic of autistic (Hutt and Hutt, 1965) and schizophrenic (Bender, 1947) children. Autistic children

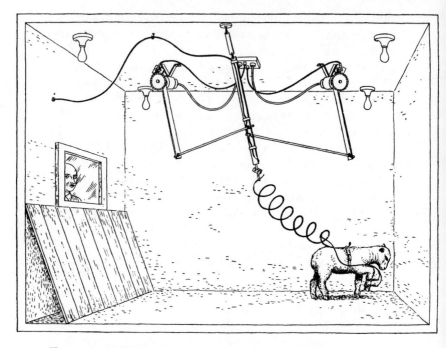

Fig. 1-12 Experimental arrangement for studying the behavior of twin lambs. *Above:* the isolated lamb; *right:* the twin placed with the mother. Both lambs received random shocks to the legs. (Reproduced from Liddell, 1954.)

seem to avoid visual novelty by their obsessive desire to maintain a familiar visual environment (Schopler, 1965), in their eye-avoidance trait, and in their preference for touch, taste, and smell rather than visual exploration. Similar symptoms have been described in 7- to 9-year-old schizophrenics.

It is interesting that in some of his aversive classical conditioning experiments with goats, Liddell (1954) noted that the presence of the mother enabled a kid to tolerate regular presentation of distressful shock stimuli. The kid and mother wandered

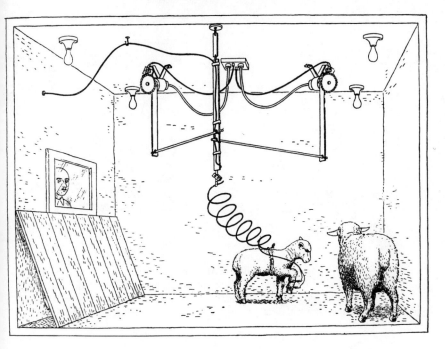

freely in a pen, but every 10 minutes the lights were turned off, and the kid received shock to the foreleg. The kid continued to move freely during the 10-minute periods, but an isolated twin kid quickly became neurotic in the situation, avoiding the center of the pen, clinging to the walls, and eventually cringing in the corner (Fig. 1-12). Such kids, unlike the mothered kid, quickly become neurotic in the classical restraining harness experiment (see p. 55).

Manipulation of reinforcement contingencies as an aversive stimulus

It is now clear that animals become very disturbed and aggressive if, when they have been conditioned to receive reinforcers

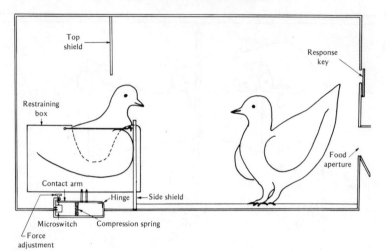

Fig. 1-13   A schematic drawing of the apparatus for measuring attack. The experimental chamber was 26 by 14 by 14 in. high. Plexiglas shields at the top and on the sides of the restraining box prevented the experimental pigeon from getting behind the target pigeon. (Reproduced from Azrin et al., 1966.)

at a certain time and of a certain magnitude for a particular response effort, they are not rewarded in the expected manner.

Azrin et al. (1966) were the first to put this form of elicited aggression under experimental control. They described a procedure in which a pigeon was alternately rewarded ten times on a continuous reinforcement schedule for pecking a key and then was given a period of extinction. At the back of a cage, a suitably restrained "target" pigeon was positioned and the attack response to it recorded (Fig. 1-13). The attacks occurred during extinction and were most frequent at the start of the extinction period. Similar behavior has been observed in the squirrel monkey, when aggression was measured by the number of bites on a piece of hose pipe placed in the animal's cage (Fig. 1-14). Hutchinson et al. (1968) observed that the withdrawal

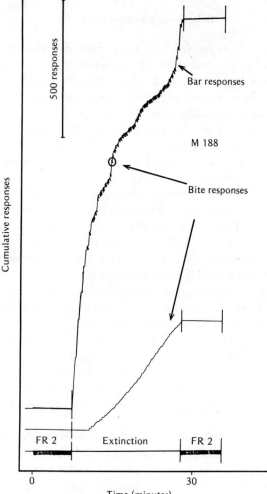

Fig. 1-14 Effect in the squirrel monkey of extinction on bar pressing and hose biting following FR 2. Bar pressing was recorded by the cumulative upward excursion of the pen in the upper curve. The response pen was reset to the base line with each reinforcement. Hose biting was recorded by the brief downward deflections of the pen in the upper curve and by the cumulative upward excursion of the pen in the center curve. Food deliveries were recorded by the brief downward movement of the pen in the lower curve. (Reproduced from Hutchinson, Azrin, and Hunt, 1968.)

of an intermittent reinforcement schedule produced more aggression than the termination of continuous reinforcement; several workers have gone on to show that fixed-ratio schedules will themselves induce aggressive responses even in the absence of any contrasting extinction period. Attack occurs with greatest frequency in the post-reinforcement pause. This has been very elegantly demonstrated by Cherek, Thompson, and Heistad (1973), who used a slightly modified Azrin apparatus. Pigeons faced two keys; pecks on one were reinforced on a 2-minute fixed-interval schedule and pecks on the other "target" key were reinforced on an FR2 schedule with access to a live target pigeon. The birds responded on the target key in the early part of the FI period and vigorously attacked the target bird when it became accessible (Fig. 1-15). Schedule-induced aggression has been observed in rats, pigeons, and monkeys.

Falk (1972) has proposed that schedule-induced aggression is similar to an abnormal drinking behavior termed schedule-induced polydipsia. If water is freely available when rats lever press for 45-mg dry food pellets on a 1-minute VI schedule, large quantities of water are consumed. During a 3.5-hour session, this can be three to four times the normal total daily intake. This does not occur with continuous reinforcement schedules but seems to appear when inter-reinforcement times exceed 30 seconds.

Falk suggests that these be called "adjunctive behaviours," which he defines as "behaviour maintained at high probability by stimuli whose reinforcing properties in the situation are derived primarily as the result of schedule parameters governing the availability of another class of reinforcers." In the experiment of Cherek et al. (1973) the reinforcing effectiveness of the opportunity to attack depended upon the presence of a schedule of food presentation. Attack no longer occurred if the animal was not exposed to the intermittent schedule of reinforcement. Adjunctive behavior resembles the "displacement activity" classically described in the ethological literature.

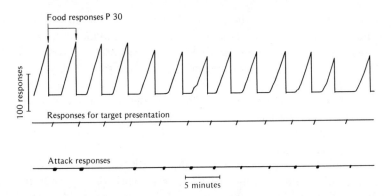

Fig. 1-15 Sample cumulative record for pigeon responding on FI 2-minute food and FR 2 target presentation schedules. Simultaneous recording of food key, target key, and attack responding are represented. Following presentation of food, the stepper pen reset to the base line (top). Attack responses are switch closures recorded when a force of at least 100 gm was exerted against the front of the restraining box (containing the target bird) by the experimental subjects during periods of fighting. The target bird was accessible for 15 seconds following completion of an FR 2 requirement on the target key. (Reproduced from Cherek et al., 1973.)

Displacement behaviors are described as occurring when certain environmental events result in the interruption of some consummatory activity in an organism under high "drive" conditioning. These are exactly the conditions that produce adjunctive aggressive behavior as defined by Falk. Aggression should not, therefore, be viewed as a behavior generated by a hypothetical internal state in the absence of eliciting stimuli, but rather as a behavior occurring in a *specific* situation—a situation in which another class of reinforcers is intermittently scheduled.

In addition to these effects of the schedule of reinforcement, sudden increases or decreases in the expected magnitude of the reward disrupt behavior. Crespi (1944) reported that if rats were trained in a runway to run to a goal box for a reinforcement of a certain size, they ran faster or slower if the size of the reward was unexpectedly increased or decreased in size. These sudden increases and decreases of ongoing behavior have been described as "behavioral contrast," and, recently, Baltzer and Weiskrantz (1970) have described a method for reliably generating these effects. Rats were trained on a 2-minute VI schedule with one pellet per reward. Then smaller and larger rewards (three or four pellets) were given on alternate daily sessions with different discriminative stimuli associated with the two conditions. After some days on the alternating procedure, daily sessions consisted of one reward condition with two brief intrusions of the other reward condition associated with the appropriate discriminative stimulus. The effects of the intrusions within each session was assessed by the quotient

$$\frac{\text{rate during intrusion} - \text{rate before intrusion}}{\text{rate during intrusion} + \text{rate before intrusion}}$$

Behavioral contrast was assessed by comparing each animal's rate on the intrusion conditions with its rate on the base-line conditions during the immediately preceding day. Larger rewards increase response rates and show positive behavioral contrast, whereas smaller rewards produce the opposite effect. The potential value of this technique, which generates behavioral states that could be likened to elation or depression, for characterizing the behavioral effects of certain drugs is mentioned later.

Experimental neurosis

In the preceding sections we have described some of the ways in which aversive stimuli disrupt ongoing behavior. The approach has been of the functional or procedural kind—not invoking unobservable variables like "fear" and "anxiety" to explain the behavioral change. This approach neglects a large body of classical experimental work on induced abnormal behavior where attempts were made to characterize the behaviors that appeared in aversive situations when a trained response was thwarted in some way. The examples to be considered concern "experimental neurosis."

Pavlovian frustration

In Pavlov's laboratory in 1921, Shenger-Krestovnikova classically conditioned a dog to salivate to a circle but not to an elipse. Finer and finer discrimination was required as the elipse was made more circular and, at the point where the dog could no longer discriminate, it became very excited and restless and so-called "neurotic" behavior emerged. Some years before, Terofeera had described similar phenomena, although their significance had not been appreciated. She conditioned salivation to an electric shock, which, after training, no longer gave rise to a strong defensive reaction. But, when she attempted to generalize the response to parts of the body that had not been originally stimulated by the shock, the defense reaction was restored and the dog showed general excitement. After Shenger-Krestovnikova's experiments, the importance of these observations became apparent to Pavlov, and the study of neurotic behavior came to dominate his experimental program. He became particularly concerned with the varying susceptibility of dogs to neurosis-inducing situations. He viewed nervous activity as a balance between excitation and inhibition and believed that dogs with a preponderance of excitation had a lower threshold for neurosis induction than those with a more strongly inhibited nervous system. Pavlov considered himself a physiologist, not a behaviorist, and this explains his concern with the interpretation of neurosis in terms of nervous activity and his lack of concern with behavioral details.

Complementary results were obtained by Liddell (1954) and his collaborators at Cornell in his classical studies of conditioned leg withdrawal in sheep and goats. The animals were placed in restraining harnesses, and front leg withdrawal was induced with electric shock. Leg withdrawal was conditioned to positive and negative stimuli, and a battery of physiological measures to assess respiration and cardiac function was taken as the animal responded. Liddell initially observed perfectly normal responses when the goat was given a limited number of trials per day, but when the number of trials in a session was increased to ten or twenty, aberrant behavior emerged. Persistent movement of the conditioned limb occurred between trials; the goat became unwilling to enter the laboratory and had to be forced onto the conditioning stand. Heartbeat and respiration became erratic. Subsequently, other modifications of the conditioning procedure were found to disrupt behavior; in order of importance they were discrimination between positive or negative stimuli, extinction of a positive conditioned response, and training on a rigid time schedule. Liddell's studies extended over many years, and he followed the social history of his subjects, their recovery, and the remission of their neurotic behavior. He reported that heartbeat in neurotic sheep is irregular under normal conditions, for example, while they are sleeping at night and, also, that they show marked frustration when mildly disturbing noises occur. Such neurotic animals also show themselves incapable of dealing with a situation of actual change in a realistic fashion. When dogs invaded the flock, it was invariably a neurotic sheep who was the victim. The animal's neurosis so damages its herd instinct that while other members of the flock escape together in one direction, the neurotic animal flees in panic in another. Clearly, both Pavlov and Liddell felt that their work on neurosis was relevant to human psychopathology.

In the next decade, Masserman (1943) took up the study of animal models of neurosis, and his interpretations had a strong psychoanalytical bias. As Broadhurst (1961) comments, "Masserman is avowedly anthropomorphic in a way which is rightly eschewed nowadays." His basic behavioral situation involved training a cat to make, in the presence of a discriminative stimulus, a box-opening response to obtain food. When the cat was well trained, box-opening attempts were accompanied by a strong puff of air and/or an electric shock. Such a procedure is essentially similar to the Geller immediate-punishment schedule. Masserman, however, was concerned with the behavior that emerged in this conflict situation rather than with the fact that box-opening was suppressed. Rating scales of enormous complexity (64 elements) were used to evaluate the neurotic profile, but it was found to be very difficult to dissociate the effect of drugs on neurosis with these methods; their value to behavioral pharmacology was summed up by Masserman and Pechtel (1956) who decided that even with the data at hand "it is impossible to state the effects of any drug on any organism without considering the latter's genetic characteristics, past experiences, biological status, and perceptions, motivations toward and evaluations of its current physical and social milieu." As Weiskrantz comments, "If this were strictly true, no pharmacology textbook could ever have been written nor any anaesthetic given with confidence" (Weiskrantz, 1968, p. 81).

We believe that terms such as "emotion," "anxiety," and "neurosis" are sometimes convenient but can easily become misleading. The safest way to measure a behavioral phenomenon is to utilize a simple operant that is a part of the constellation but can be quantified. This explains our preoccupation in the earlier parts of this chapter with the parametric studies of how aversive stimuli change specified elements of conditioned or unconditioned behavior.

2 | Basic Neuropharmacology

SOME BASIC PHARMACOLOGICAL PRINCIPLES

What is a drug?

A drug is any substance that can interact with a biological system. The neuropharmacologist's concern is with the large number of drugs that affect nervous tissue. For the purpose of this book, in which our main objective is to consider the actions of those drugs that interact with the nervous system to produce changes in behavior, the focus of attention will clearly be even more restricted. Thus we will not be considering the many drugs that specifically interact with the central nervous system of mammals to produce anesthesia (anesthetics), sleep (hypnotics), or relief from pain (analgesics) or drugs used to combat epileptic conditions (anticonvulsants). Nor will we deal in any detail with those drugs whose primary site of action is the peripheral motor, sensory, or autonomic nervous systems, such as local anesthetics and ganglion-blocking drugs. Our interest is primarily in the drugs that affect mood and behavior, the so-called psychotropic drugs.

How drugs work and how their effects are measured

Most drugs interact in a specific manner with target sites in biological systems; such sites are pharmacologically defined as DRUG

RECEPTORS. The drug-receptor interaction does not usually involve a covalent chemical linkage of the drug to the receptor, but rather a weaker interaction whereby the drug because of its particular shape and charge distribution can bind reversibly to a specific chemical site on the receptor and, in so doing, change the physiological reactivity of the receptor. The receptor, for example, may be an enzyme, and the drug may act to inhibit its activity. Alternatively, drug receptors may be specific membrane proteins in such excitable tissues as nerve or muscle, in which the drug-receptor interaction leads to a change in membrane permeability that, in turn, excites or inhibits the excitable cell. Not all drugs act by way of such specific receptor interactions; for example, many anesthetic drugs change the electric properties of nerves by dissolving in the lipoprotein membranes of such cells; this produces an over-all change in the physiochemical properties of the membranes thus inhibiting excitation. The great majority of drugs, however, have more specific receptor interactions.

These drugs produce biological responses that are graded according to the amount of drug administered (DOSE). Such dose-response relationships are most conveniently plotted as biological response (on a linear scale) against log of dose, to yield an S-shaped (sigmoid) LOG DOSE-RESPONSE CURVE (Fig. 2-1). This is by no means the only way of expressing drug responses, but it has several advantages over other graphical expressions. It allows us to depict drug responses over a wide range of doses, since the dosage scale is compressed by the log conversion. It is also found that, though the log dose-response is a sigmoid curve, an important portion of it (about 30 to 70% of the maximum response) approximates a straight line, thus making it possible to quantify and compare data in this dose-response range. Furthermore, a series of different drugs that produce the same response by interacting by a common receptor mechanism will give a series of parallel log dose-response curves. In such a series, the curve for the drug that interacts most strongly with the receptor

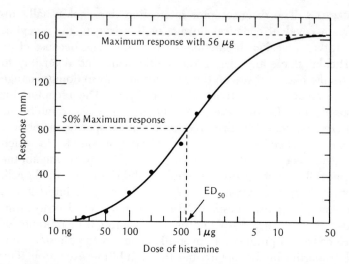

Fig. 2-1 Log dose-response curve for histamine acting on guinea pig ileum in an organ bath. Response magnitude (mm) is proportional to contraction of the ileum. Histamine dose added to a constant volume bath is shown on a logarithmic scale. (From Goldstein, Aranow, and Kalman, 1969.)

will appear to the left of the others, since lower doses will be needed to produce the biological response. The POTENCY of drugs can thus be compared. The potency of a drug is often expressed as the dose required to produce one-half of the maximum response the drug is capable of eliciting; this is the ED_{50}. The shape of the log dose-response curve reflects the nature of the drug-receptor interaction. This interaction is analogous to the binding of substrate molecules to an enzyme. It is an equilibrium reaction, and the proportion of receptors occupied by the drug will depend on the affinity of the drug molecules for the receptors and the drug concentration at the level of the receptors. Since the number of receptor sites in a given tissue is finite, the drug-receptor interaction is a saturable relationship in which increasing the drug concentration (or dose) beyond a certain point cannot lead to further increase in drug binding, since all available receptors, or at least all those needed to produce a maximum biological response, are occupied.

Some drugs, known as AGONISTS, produce a direct measurable response by interacting with receptors, but other types of drugs alter the response normally elicited from the interaction of agonists with their receptors. Thus, ANTAGONIST drugs block the responses normally elicited by agonists. A simple, competitive antagonist, as the name implies, competes with an agonist drug for binding to the receptor sites. When receptor sites are occupied by the antagonist molecules, no response is produced, and the sites are not available to the agonist. Such competitive antagonism can be overcome, however, if the dose of agonist is increased. The actions of a competitive antagonist thus show up as a shift to the right in the log dose-response curve of the agonist drug (Fig. 2-2A). Non-competitive antagonists block receptors in a way that cannot be overcome by increasing the agonist dose. The agonist log dose-response curve is again shifted to the right, but the maximum response is also depressed by the antagonist (Fig. 2-2B). Other drugs may increase the potency of an agonist, a phenomenon known as POTENTIATION which involves a shift in the agonist log dose-response curve to the left. Such potentiation is usually a consequence of more agonist drug being made available to interact with its receptors, rather than of any fundamental change in the properties of the receptors. Potentiation may occur, for example, by inhibiting the mechanisms normally responsible for removing an agonist from the environment of its receptors by metabolism or by tissue uptake mechanisms.

The use of log dose-response curves to assess the effects of drugs on behavior is no less desirable than in any other branch of pharmacology. Such a systematic approach allows us to compare the potencies of different drugs in a series of related compounds; at the same time it indicates whether these drugs act by way of a common mechanism. It also allows us to determine

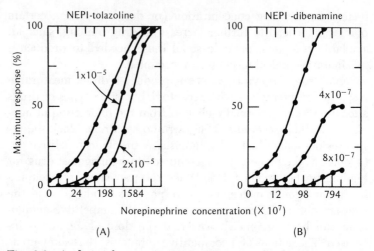

Fig. 2-2   Analysis of receptor antagonist actions by log dose-response curves. Isolated cat spleen strips stimulated by norepinephrine (NEPI) at various concentrations at low and high concentrations of a competitive antagonists; (A) tolazoline, or a non-competitive antagonist; (B) dibenamine. (From Goldstein, Aranow, and Kalman, 1969.)

agonist/antagonist relationships and to compare the properties of drug receptors in the brain with receptors in the peripheral nervous system. There are several difficulties, however, in applying such an analysis to the effects of drugs on behavior. Classically, drug-receptor interactions are studied with simple isolated tissue systems (see Figs. 2-1 and 2-2), in which the concentration of drug to which the receptors are exposed is known and easily controllable and in which the drug interacts with only one type of receptor to produce a single type of response. Matters are never this simple in behavioral pharmacology. Behavioral responses are clearly of a far more complex nature than the contraction of a piece of smooth muscle in an organ bath. A behavioral response cannot always be easily quantified and measured on a linear scale, on which the magnitude of the response di-

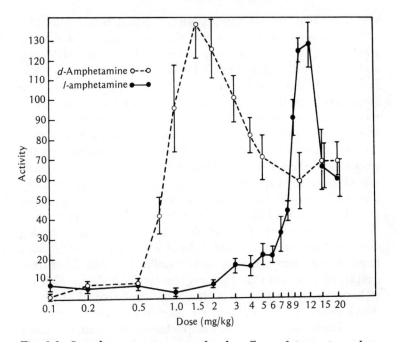

Fig. 2-3 Log dose-response curves for the effects of increasing subcutaneous doses of *d*- and *l*-amphetamine on locomotor activity in rats pretreated with iproniazid (150 mg/kg, i.p.) 16 hours earlier. Rats were placed in individual photocell activity cages, and locomotor activity was measured as the number of interruption of the photocell beam in a 30-minute session. Each point is the mean and standard error for six determinations. (From Taylor and Snyder, 1971.)

rectly reflects the drug-receptor interaction. Apart from difficulties of measurement, one particular behavioral response may have complex effects on other behavioral responses, which, in turn, modify the response being measured; alternatively, the drug-receptor interaction may produce more than one type of response. Drugs often have multiple actions on different receptors in the brain, leading to a complex series of behavioral consequences that are not easily analyzed. Apart from these difficulties, there is the problem that the concentration of drug to which receptors in the brain are exposed is usually not known and cannot easily be controlled. For example, agonist drugs may have widely different potencies in eliciting a given behavioral response not because of any real difference in their potencies at receptor sites in the brain, but simply because some drugs penetrate more readily into the brain from the bloodstream than others. This problem is discussed in more detail below. Lest the reader be dismayed by the difficulties of the quantitative analysis of behavioral responses to drugs, it should be pointed out that such analysis is often possible, and the results can be valuable. For example, Fig. 2-3 shows an analysis and comparison of the motor stimulant effects of d- and l-amphetamine. The log dose-response curves are conventional in the sense that the lines from the two drugs are essentially parallel, but they differ from simpler responses in that the curves do not show simple plateaus at high doses of either drug, but rather bell-shaped curves in which the response falls off at very high doses. The result, however, clearly indicates that d-amphetamine is about ten times more potent than l-amphetamine in stimulating locomotor activity in the rat.

The penetration of drugs into the central nervous system after peripheral administration

Drugs are most often administered systemically. This may be done by mouth (PER OS, P.O.) or by injection into the peritoneal cavity (INTRAPERITONEALLY, I.P.), into a large muscle (INTRAMUSCULARLY, I.M.), under the skin (SUBCUTANEOUSLY, S.C.), or into the bloodstream, usually by injection into a vein (INTRAVENOUSLY, I.V.). In all of these cases, the drug is distributed throughout the various tissues of the body after entering the bloodstream. The amount of drug entering peripheral tissues will depend on the rate at which blood flows through these tissues and on the ease with which the drug can escape from the bloodstream to enter the tissues. Most drugs escape readily from small blood vessels and equilibrate rapidly with the extracellular fluid space of peripheral tissues, from which a drug may then act on receptors on the external surfaces of cell membranes or may penetrate into the cells. The penetration of drugs from the blood into the central nervous system (CNS), however, is a special case. Drugs may enter the CNS either by direct penetration into the brain or spinal cord through brain capillaries or they may first enter the cerebrospinal fluid (CSF) from the blood and thence into the CNS tissue. In either case, the rate of penetration for most drugs is relatively slow compared to the rate of distribution of drugs into peripheral tissues. The brain has a very high blood flow, about 0.5 ml/gm/minute compared with about 0.05 ml/gm/minute in resting muscle, but drugs and other substances escape from the brain capillaries far less readily than from the capillaries in most other tissues. This is partly due to the special nature of the brain capillary walls, which lack the pores or fenestrations found in peripheral blood vessels. Substances passing out of brain capillary vessels have thus to pass through the endothelial cells of which the capillary wall is composed, rather than simply through the pores in the wall. In addition, the brain capillaries are wrapped tightly in a sheath of glial tissue made up of the processes of numerous astrocytes. This glial sheath is closely apposed to the surface of the capillaries and covers more than 80% of the exterior of the capillary. Finally, the CNS differs from most peripheral organs in that its cellular elements (neurons and glial cells) are tightly packed together, with only very small and tortuous clefts of extracellular space between them. Estimates of the volume of extracellular space indicate that it may be as little as 5-15% of the brain volume, compared with the 20-40% found in most other tissues. These unique anatomical features lead to a situation in which drugs and other water-soluble substances do not readily penetrate into the brain from the bloodstream.

Most water-soluble substances penetrate the brain only after they have crossed the cell barriers of the capillary endothelium and its surrounding glial sheath, a process that is much slower than penetration through fenestrated capillaries into the extracellular space of the peripheral tissues. This unique relationship between blood supply and brain tissue has led to the concept of a BLOOD-BRAIN BARRIER, which describes the relatively slow penetration of many substances from blood into brain. The term "barrier," however, is now generally accepted as a somewhat misleading description of the phenomenon, since there is probably no single anatomical feature that can be described as a barrier. Furthermore, the phenomenon is not so much that there is an absolute barrier to the penetration of substances into the brain, but rather that the *rate* of penetration is in general slower for brain than for most other tissues.

Penetration of drugs into the CSF occurs either by passage through the brain capillaries into the extracellular fluid of the brain—with which the CSF fairly readily equilibrates—or by passage through the blood vessels of the choroid plexus, the specialized, highly vascular structure in the ventricular system from which CSF is formed. In either case, the penetration of drugs into the CSF usually occurs no more readily than into the brain tissue. Once drugs have entered the CSF, however, they may leave the brain only slowly, since the CSF equilibrates only slowly with other body fluids.

The brain is not homogeneous in its blood-tissue permeability properties. Some regions of the CNS appear to lack any blood-brain barrier, and drugs and other substances penetrate readily; these include the pineal gland, the posterior lobe of the pituitary gland, and the area postrema, a small region situated on the roof of the fourth ventricle in the brain stem, which contains the chemoreceptors involved in the control of vomiting. The rate of penetration of drugs into other brain regions is not uniform. Regional blood flow varies considerably, with rates as high as 2.0 ml/gm/minute in some cortical gray matter and as low as 0.2 ml/gm/minute in most white matter. Consequently the distribution of drugs in the CNS is not even, and higher drug concentrations are reached—at least for short periods of time after drug administration—in regions in which gray matter predominates.

Since the "blood-brain barrier" poses such important problems for the interpretation of drug action on the CNS, it is worth considering some of the properties of drug molecules that are important in determining the rate at which they penetrate into the CNS after peripheral administration. Because of the cellular barriers involved in the penetration of drugs into the CNS from the bloodstream, the rules governing the permeability characteristics of the blood-brain barrier are similar to those governing the penetration of drugs or other substances across cell membranes, rather than through the usual capillary fenestrations in other tissues. The general principles involved are quite well understood and can be summarized as follows:

Binding to plasma proteins

Since only free drug molecules are available for passage across cell membranes, the extent of drug molecule binding to plasma proteins can be important. This binding reduces the plasma concentration of drug available for entry into the brain. In many cases, the proportion of circulating drug bound in this way can be very high; values of more than 90% are not uncommon.

Ionization of charged groups

Many drugs have ionizable groups, usually a weak acid or base, so that the ionization is incomplete at physiological pH values. The degree of ionization of such groups at physiological pH is a vital factor in drug penetration, since the permeability of cell membranes to the electrically charged ionized form of the molecule is usually very low compared to the much higher permeability of the same compound in the un-ionized (electrically neutral) form. The extent of ionization of these weakly acidic or basic groups on drug molecules at physiological pH is, in turn, determined by the chemical nature of the remainder of the drug molecule and can be estimated from the drug's pK value, the pH at which 50% of the drug molecules exist in the ionized form.

The importance of ionization in determining the penetration of substances from the blood into the brain is illustrated by the complete lack of penetration of such circulating organic amines as epinephrine (E), norepinephrine (NE), dopamine (DA), and acetylcholine (ACh) (see below). The pK of these substances is in the alkaline range, so that at physiological pH they exist almost entirely in the ionized form, with a positive electric charge. As an example, the CNS action of the cholinergic-blocking drugs, atropine, and its close analogue methylatropine can be compared (Fig. 2-13). These two drugs are of comparable potency in antagonizing cholinergic receptors in peripheral tissue, but the potency of atropine is many times that of its methyl analogue in the CNS. This is explained by the relative lack of penetration of methyl atropine into the CNS, the methyl substituent converting the neutral drug atropine into a positively charged quaternary nitrogen compound.

Lipid solubility

The solubility of a drug in lipid is also of major importance in determining its rate of penetration into the CNS. Drugs that are quite soluble in lipid penetrate lipoprotein cell membranes far more readily than drugs that are relatively insoluble. Lipid solubility is indicated by the partition coefficient of the substance between an organic solvent (such as benzene or heptane) and water, here, the proportion of drug in the water and in the organic solvent phase as measured after equilibrium has been reached.

The role of these various factors in determining the rate of penetration of drugs into the CNS is illustrated by the results listed in Table 2-1, which compares the extent of protein bind-

TABLE 2-1

CORRELATION OF PHYSICAL PROPERTIES OF DRUGS WITH THEIR RATES
OF PENETRATION INTO THE CEREBROSPINAL FLUID

Drug	Fraction bound to plasma protein*	Fraction un-ionized*	Partition coefficient n-heptane/ water of un-ionized form	CSF penetration†
Thiopental	0.75	0.61	3.30	1.4
Aniline	0.15	0.99	1.10	1.7
Pentobarbital	0.40	0.83	0.05	4.0
Barbital	0.02	0.56	0.002	27.0
Mecamylamine	0.20	0.02	400.0	32.0
Salicylic acid	0.40	0.004	0.12	112.0

(Modified from Goldstein, Aranow, and Kalman, 1969.)

* At pH 7.4.

† CSF penetration rates were recorded in dogs by measuring drug
concentration in CSF at various times after drug administration.
Results are expressed as the half-time (minutes) taken for the CSF
concentration of drug to equilibrate with that in plasma.

ing, ionization, and lipid solubility of various drugs with the
rates of penetration measured experimentally by the analysis of
samples of CSF taken at various times after drug administration.
Such drugs as thiopental and aniline penetrate into the CNS very
rapidly because they are largely un-ionized at plasma pH and are
soluble in lipids. Pentobarbital is much less soluble in lipid
than is thiopental and penetrates more slowly. This correlates
well with the almost immediate induction of anesthesia after
an intravenous administration of thiopental, compared with the
relatively slow induction after pentobarbital. Salicylic acid and
mecamylamine are examples of drugs that penetrate into the
CNS only poorly because they are very largely ionized at physiological pH. Though un-ionized mecamylamine is relatively solu-

ble in lipid, the ionized form is not, and CSF penetration occurs only slowly.

Alternative methods of administering drugs to avoid the blood-brain barrier

Because of the relatively poor penetration of many drugs into the brain following systemic administration, a number of alternative approaches have been devised to circumvent this problem. The most direct approach is to administer the drug directly into the brain, and a number of ways of doing this are available. One can inject or infuse a solution containing drug into the CSF and observe its effects on behavior. To avoid performing the injection in an anesthetized animal, such administrations are often made through small tubes (cannulae) that have been surgically implanted under anesthesia. Such permanently implanted cannulae are easily fitted through the skull of such small laboratory animals as the rat. Drug solutions injected into the CSF rapidly diffuse through the ventricular system, and drugs administered in this way gain ready access to many brain regions; there are, however, regional differences in the permeability of the lining of the ventricles, and some brain structures, which lie far away from the ventricular surfaces, may not be so readily exposed to the injected drug. In larger animals, several cannulae can be implanted in different parts of the ventricular system of the brain, so that drug solutions may be perfused through restricted areas of the CSF, thus exposing selected brain regions only. An even more selective exposure of brain regions to drugs is achieved by the micro-injection of very small volumes of drug solution into a local region of brain tissue itself. This is done through very fine diameter needles or cannulae, the tips of which are precisely located in the brain by implantation with the aid of a stereotaxic apparatus and an appropriate brain atlas. Unless very small volumes are injected (less than 1 μl), however, the injected substance may still spread to regions up to 1 mm or more from the site of injection—a relatively large distance in such animals as mice and rats whose brains are quite small. The spread of the injected drug should ideally be determined by using radioactively labeled drug for test injections and examining the distribution of radioactivity at various times after injection.

An even more precise localization of administered drug can be achieved by the ejection of very small amounts of the drug from the tips of fine glass microelectrodes, using the passage of electric current through the electrode to move the charged drug molecules by iontophoresis. This technique has proved useful for studying the responses of single neurons in the CNS to a variety of test substances (see p. 93), but it seems unlikely to be of value for behavioral studies, since in order to evoke a measurable change in behavior it would probably be necessary to influence more than a small number of neurons. Also, the technique can be applied only to fully anesthetized animals at present.

At first glance, it might seem that the intracerebral administration of drugs would be the method of choice for studying drug actions on the CNS, since it avoids many of the difficulties outlined. One might think that this offers a method whereby the dose of drug applied to the brain could be precisely controlled and that a series of related drugs could thus be subjected to quantitative pharmacological analysis to assess their potencies in eliciting various forms of behavior. Although this may occasionally be possible, there are unfortunately a number of difficulties. The most important of these is that when drugs are administered intracerebrally they tend to leave the brain rather rapidly, and different drugs will leave at different rates. The rate at which substances leave the brain, largely by entrance into the bloodstream, is determined by factors similar to those previously described for the entry of substances from blood to brain. Thus, small uncharged molecules, which are very soluble in lipid, will disappear very rapidly, whereas water-soluble acids or bases may persist a much longer period of time. All substances administered in this way, however, will tend to escape relatively rapidly because the injection of a small amount of material into the brain or CSF means that there is always a large concentration gradient between the brain and the peripheral tissue, especially the relatively large volume of drug-free blood. Nevertheless, this technique has proved useful, particularly for drugs that hardly penetrate into the brain after systemic administration; these include the transmitter amines and amino acids, NE, DA, ACh, gamma-aminobutyric acid (GABA), and related compounds.

Another way of circumventing the blood-brain barrier is to observe the behavioral effects of systemically administered drugs in very young animals, in which the blood-brain barrier is not yet developed. For example, most substances penetrate readily into the CNS from the bloodstream in chicks, in which the normal blood-brain barrier is not fully developed until about 1 week after hatching. In mammals, such as the rat, a similar situation exists for the first few days after birth. This phenomenon has proved valuable in studying the CNS activity of otherwise impermeant substances, but this approach is, of course, limited by the fact that the brain is still highly immature in such young animals. They thus have neither the neuropharmacological nor the behavioral repertoire of the adult, and behavioral responses to drugs may not reflect the normal responses of the mature CNS.

A final maneuver is to achieve exposure of the CNS to a drug by administering a precursor substance that penetrates into the CNS more readily than the drug itself and can be converted to the desired drug after it has entered the CNS. In the case of the transmitter amines, DA and 5-HT, for example, the precursor amino acids L-dopa and L-5-hydroxytryptophan enter the CNS after systemic administration, whereas the amines hardly penetrate the CNS. The amino acids are readily converted in the brain to the amines by aromatic amino acid decarboxylase. The amino acids probably enter the brain by way of special membrane transport systems, which the brain uses to obtain such substances as glucose or amino acids from the bloodstream. This approach has many virtues. In the examples cited above, the precursor substances themselves are virtually devoid of pharmacological activity and can be used in relatively large doses to load the CNS with active metabolites. Other examples include the metabolic conversion of the inactive drug chloral hydrate into the active CNS depressant trichlorethanol and the conversion of the weak cholinergic agonist tremorine into the more active oxotremorine (Fig. 2-13). Unfortunately, this approach is limited by the availability of suitable precursors that penetrate readily into the CNS.

Drug metabolism

Most drugs are metabolized in the body, and most of their metabolic products are both pharmacologically less active than the parent drug and more readily excreted. Generally, metabolism leads to a product that is more highly ionized than the parent drug. This product is then less readily reabsorbed from the renal tubules and is excreted more rapidly in the urine. By contrast, un-ionized, lipid-soluble substances readily diffuse back into the blood after filtration in the kidneys are thus less rapidly excreted in the urine. Drugs may be combined with such highly ionized substances as glucuronic acid, sulfate ions, and acetate, thus facilitating their excretion.

A wide variety of enzymes and many different types of chemical transformation are involved in drug metabolism, and a large literature on the subject now exists. The reactions usually involve oxidation, reduction, or hydrolysis. The major site of drug metabolism is the liver, but other sites include the kidneys, lungs, and blood plasma; some metabolism may occur within the CNS. An important series of enzymes involved in the metabolism of drugs is located in the membrane of the endoplasmic reticulum of the liver.

TABLE 2-2

SPECIES DIFFERENCES IN METABOLISM OF HEXOBARBITAL; CHANGES
WITH AGE

Species	Average sleeping time (minutes)	Hexobarbital half-life in plasma (minutes)	Liver enzyme activity (μg/gm hour^{-1})
Mice	12 ± 8	19±7	598 ± 184
Rabbits	49 ± 12	60 ± 11	196 ± 28
Rats	90 ± 15	140 ± 54	134 ± 51
Dogs	315 ± 105	260 ± 20	36 ± 30

(Hexobarbital dose in all species except dog, 100 mg/kg;
dog, 50 mg/kg)

	Average sleeping time (minutes)	Injected drug metabolized in 3 hours (%)	Liver enzyme activity (% added drug metabolized per hour)
Mice:			
1-day-old	360	0	0
7-day-old	107 ± 26	11-25	2.5-3.5
21-day-old	27 ± 11	21-33	13-21
Adult	5	–	28-39

(Hexobarbital dose, 10 mg/kg)

(From Goldstein, Aranow, and Kalman, 1969.)

An important feature of the hepatic metabolizing enzymes is
that the amount of these enzymes present in the liver can increase
if the drugs that are metabolized by them are administered repeatedly. The repeated administration of such barbiturates as
pentobarbital or phenobarbital, for example, gradually leads to

an increase in the hepatic enzymes responsible for degrading these drugs. The result is that they are more rapidly degraded, and their action is progressively diminished upon repeated administration. Since the hepatic enzymes are relatively nonspecific, the metabolism of one drug may be influenced by prior administration of any other drug that can increase the enzymatic machinery of the liver. Differences in the activity of hepatic drug-metabolizing enzymes between different species, between male and female animals of the same species, or between individuals of different ages may also be important in determining the pharmacological response to drugs. These factors are illustrated in Table 2-2, for the sedative hexobarbital, for which the rate of drug metabolism is easily related to pharmacological effects, as measured by the average duration of sleep induced by the drug.

Tolerance and physical dependence

DRUG TOLERANCE is the term used to describe the diminished responsiveness of animals or man to a drug after previous administration of the drug or some related substance. PHYSICAL DEPENDENCE, sometimes associated with tolerance, is the term used to describe a state in which, after repeated drug administration, the organism may actually require the presence of the drug for normal functioning. Such a state of dependence or addiction is revealed by withdrawing the drug, which elicits a variety of physiological disturbances known collectively as the WITHDRAWAL SYNDROME. Virtually all of the effects of the withdrawal syndrome are rapidly terminated if the drug is re-administered.

Tolerance and dependence are all too common features of psychoactive drug use. They arise by mechanisms that are largely unknown. One important mechanism that is fairly well understood is the induction of drug-metabolizing enzymes on repeated drug administration. At the least, this phenomenon can account for an important component of the tolerance that develops to such drugs as hexobarbital and pentobarbital upon repeated administration. Tolerance in such cases is due to an increased rate of metabolism of the administered drug, so that for a given dose the duration of effective exposure of the tissues to the active drug progressively diminishes as administration is continued. Even with the barbiturates, other less well understood mechanisms are involved in the development of tolerance. Rats given barbiturates repeatedly show progressively shorter periods of anesthesia following drug administration. That this cannot simply be due to a more rapid rate of drug metabolism is shown by the finding that the concentration of free drug in the brain at the time the animals wake up from the anesthesia progressively increases with repeated doses. Thus, the animals' threshold for anesthesia gradually increases. This is due to some cellular adaptation in the brain, whereby the receptors responsible for the drug action become less sensitive to the drug—a phenomenon sometimes called CELLULAR TOLERANCE.

Although tolerance develops to many psychoactive drugs, this is not always accompanied by the development of physical dependence. For example, tolerance to the hallucinogenic effects of lysergic acid diethylamide (LSD) develops rapidly in man, but there is no evidence of physical dependence. A similar situation holds for the amphetamines and the cannabis alkaloids. On the other hand, man and animals clearly show the development of tolerance and physical dependence after prolonged administration of alcohol, barbiturates, meprobamate, or the opium alkaloids. The latter group of drugs includes morphine, heroin, levorphanol, meperidine, and methadone (see p. 205). These drugs produce striking degrees of tolerance and dependence in animals and in man. Morphine addicts have been known to take daily doses of several grams, whereas such doses would almost certainly prove lethal to a naive subject. Rodents can be made tolerant to morphine by repeated administration of this or a related drug over a period of a few days (Fig. 2-4). The use of

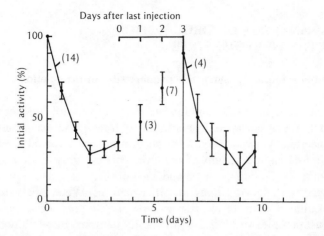

Fig. 2-4 Development of tolerance to morphine in mice. The effects of repeated doses of morphine (20 mg/kg every 16 hours) in stimulating running activity (measured with photocell cages) rapidly diminish. After six doses, drug treatment was stopped and some animals were tested with a single dose of morphine 1, 2 or 3 days later; note the reversal of tolerance during this period. When regular treatment was started again, tolerance again developed in a similar manner. (From Goldstein and Sheehan, 1969.)

behavioral techniques to assess the development of tolerance and dependence to the narcotic drugs in animals will be discussed in more detail in Chapter 4.

Tolerance and dependence remain major problems in the use of many psychoactive drugs by man; they also present a formidable challenge to pharmacologists to understand the basic cellular mechanisms underlying these striking phenomena. Almost certainly, cellular changes in the biosynthesis of receptor molecules or of enzymes involved in the synthesis or breakdown of neurotransmitters or hormones are provoked by long-term drug administration, but the precise nature of these changes remains unknown.

THE ANALYSIS OF DRUG ACTION
ON THE NERVOUS SYSTEM

The neuron and the synapse—primary sites of drug action

The mammalian brain contains an incredibly complex collection of millions of nerve cells (neurons) with many billions of interconnections between them. The sheer numbers involved are difficult to imagine: 1 gm of cerebral cortical gray matter may contain 200 million neurons, and each of these on average makes contact with several thousand other neurons. When brain tissue is examined with an electron microscope, it presents an image of vast complexity (Fig. 2-5) including neurons, their many thin axonal and dendritic processes, and the specialized zones of contact between neurons known as synapses. Virtually all of the remaining space in the tissue is filled with the cytoplasm of the supporting cells, or neuroglia, of which there are several distinct varieties.

Although some synapses operate by direct electric communication between neurons, the great majority of synaptic contacts involve a process of chemical transmission, in which the arrival of a nerve impulse or an action potential at the terminal region of an axonal process leads to the release of a minute amount of chemical transmitter. This chemical messenger rapidly diffuses across the narrow cleft filled with extracellular fluid, that separates the nerve terminal from the dendrite or cell body of the neuron with which it communicates (the postsynaptic cell). The transmitter then acts upon specialized receptor sites on the surface of the postsynaptic cell to trigger a rapid and short-lasting change in the permeability of the cell membrane. Depending on which transmitter substance and which type of receptor site are involved, this change in membrane permeability may either excite or inhibit the firing of action potentials by the postsynaptic cell. Excitation is usually accompanied by an in-

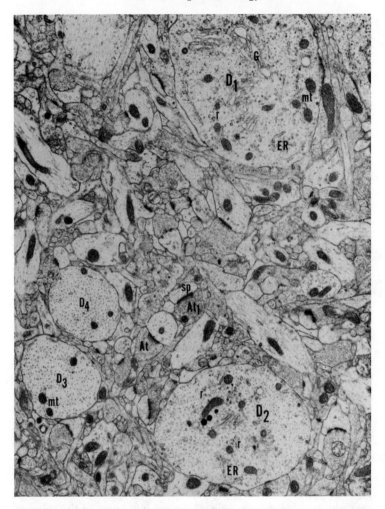

Fig. 2-5   Electron micrograph of the parietal cortex of the rat, layers II and III. The section is taken parallel to the surface of the cortex so that several apical dendrites (D_1-D_4) are seen in cross section. Note the tight packing of the neuropil. Sections through the base of dendrites contain Golgi apparatus (G), mitochondria (mt), endoplasmic reticulum (ER), ribosomes (r), and microtubules in their cytoplasm. Dendritic spines (sp) with axon terminals (At) synapsing on them can also be seen. Magnification, X 15,000. (From Peters, 1970.)

crease in the permeability of the cell membrane to extracellular, positively charged ions, such as sodium, which then enters rapidly and momentarily depolarizes the postsynaptic cell. This, in turn, leads to the firing of a propagated action potential by the cell. Inhibitory synaptic transmission, however, is probably just as common as excitatory transmission in the mammalian CNS and is certainly just as important for the integrative functions of the neuronal network of the CNS, which would otherwise be in an uncontrolled and meaningless state of activity because of the rich interconnections between neurons. Inhibition is often brought about by a selective increase in the ionic permeability of the postsynaptic cell membrane to a negatively charged ion, such as chloride, which then enters to cause a hyperpolarization of the cell, making it relatively refractive to firing. In the mammalian CNS, most neurons receive a large number of synaptic inputs; large neurons in the cerebral cortex may have as many as 3000 to 4000 per cell. The inputs are both excitatory and inhibitory, so the activity of the cell from moment to moment is governed by the balance of these inputs. The neuron acts to integrate the excitatory and inhibitory synaptic inputs, which determine the rate of firing.

Although this simplified account might suggest that the CNS could function with only two transmitter substances—one for excitation and one for inhibition—this is not the case. At least seven different transmitter substances are known in synaptic transmission in the mammalian CNS, and more probably remain to be discovered. The reason for this multiplicity of transmitters is not clear, but it may represent a mechanism for increasing the information content of the message transmitted across a synaptic junction, which may not simply be an "on" or "off" switch but may also involve more subtle long-term influences of the released transmitter on the postsynaptic cells. A multiplicity of transmitters may, in addition, control the firing of postsynaptic cells more subtly, since the precise excitatory or inhibitory responses evoked by different transmitters are not the same, some produc-

TABLE 2-3

NEUROTRANSMITTER SUBSTANCES

Transmitter	Synonyms	Abbreviation
Acetylcholine	—	ACh
Dopamine	—	DA
Gamma aminobutyric acid	—	GABA
Glutamic acid	—	Glu
Glycine	—	Gly
5-Hydroxytryptamine	Serotonin	5-HT
Norepinephrine	Noradrenaline	NE
	Arterenol	

ing, for example, inhibitory responses of very short duration (fractions of a millisecond), whereas others produce an inhibitory response of much longer duration (hundreds of milliseconds). The current list of substances known to act as transmitter substances is given in Table 2-3; all of them are small, water-soluble molecules that diffuse easily. All contain amine groups that are ionized at physiological pH, and the amino acid transmitters contain one or more carboxylic acid groups that are also ionized at physiological pH. Two of these substances, acetylcholine (ACh) and norepinephrine (NE) exist in the peripheral nervous system where they also act as transmitters, in this case mainly between neurons and a variety of effector tissues innervated by these neurons. Acetylcholine, for example, is the transmitter responsible for eliciting contraction from skeletal muscles in response to activity in the motor nerves innervating them. This amine is also released from both pre- and post-ganglionic parasympathetic nerves, mediating transmission between these two neurons in parasympathetic ganglia and between postganglionic parasympathetic nerves and the various muscle and glandular tissues of the viscera they innervate. Norepinephrine is the transmitter released by postganglionic neurons of the sympathetic nervous system; it elicits responses from the muscle and glandular tissues innervated by this system including heart muscle and the smooth muscle of the blood vessels, intestine, and urogenital system. The transmission of impulses from preganglionic sympathetic neurons to the NE-containing postganglionic neurons again involves ACh release from the preganglionic nerve terminals in sympathetic ganglia. Because ACh and NE were the first transmitters to be discovered, and because they can be studied easily in the readily accessible effector junctions and ganglia of the peripheral motor and autonomic nervous systems, a great deal of information is available about these two substances. The way in which they act on postsynaptic cells, the biochemistry of the mechanisms involved in their metabolism, release, and inactivation, and the actions of drugs on these systems are far better understood than are those for any of the other more recently discovered CNS transmitters. Fortunately, most of the knowledge gained from studies of cholinergic (acetylcholine) and adrenergic (catecholamine) mechanisms in the peripheral nervous system can be applied to those neuronal systems in the CNS that use these transmitters. Studies of such mechanisms for other CNS transmitters, however, have proved far more difficult because synapses in the brain and spinal cord are far less accessible for experimental analysis than are peripheral synapses. The methods that have been developed for such studies will be outlined below.

Because many drugs that alter CNS function out primarily at the synaptic level, the basic design and properties of synaptic junctions are worth considering in more detail. A typical CNS synapse is shown as it appears under the electron microscope in Fig. 2-6, and in diagrammatic form in Fig. 2-7. The synapse is an area of specialized contact between two cellular elements—the presynaptic nerve terminal and a small area of the surface of the postsynaptic cell. The presynaptic element is often a "swollen" terminal of one of the fine branches of the axons of the presynaptic neuron. In some neurons, such synaptic swellings or *boutons* are not restricted to the axon terminals but occur at many re-

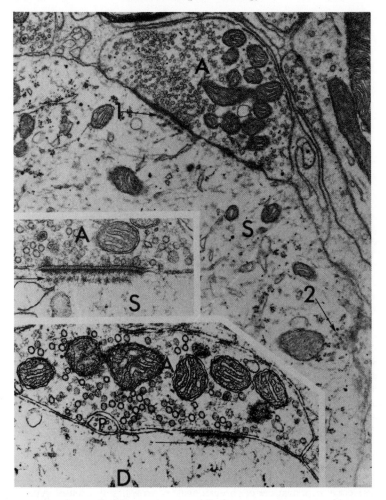

Fig. 2-6 Electron micrographs of synapses in cat oculomotor nucleus. A presynaptic terminal (A) makes synaptic contact with a large cell body (S), and under this synapse are a number of postsynaptic dense bodies (1). The insets show a similar synapse on a cell body and on a dendrite (D). Magnification, X 30,000 (insets, X 50,000). (From Pappas and Waxman, 1972.)

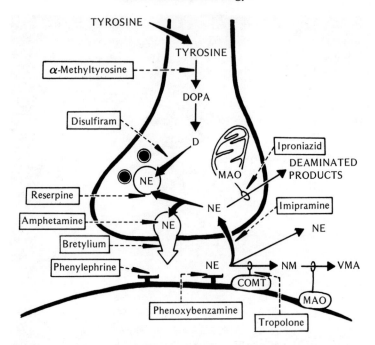

Fig. 2-7 A diagrammatic scheme indicating the multiple sites of drug action at a noradrenergic synapse. Some of the drugs that alter adrenergic transmission are shown; details of these actions are discussed in the text. COMT, catechol-O-methyl transferase; MAO, monoamine oxidase; NE, norepinephrine (noradrenaline); NM, normetanephrine; VMA, 3-methoxy, 4-hydroxymendelic acid; DOPA, 3,4-dihydroxyphenylalamine. (From Rech and Moore, 1971.)

gions along the course of the axon, so that the nerve fiber has a varicose appearance; each varicosity represents an area of synaptic contact. Each bouton can thus make contact with a large number of postsynaptic cells. This type of terminal arrangement is characteristic of neurons using NE, DA, and 5-HT as transmitters. The bouton or varicosity contains a store of the transmitter, usually concentrated within the numerous small membrane-enclosed spherical bodies known as SYNAPTIC VESICLES, which are found in abundance in the cytoplasm of the presynaptic axon. The cytoplasm of the bouton also contains mitochondria, all of the enzymes needed for energy metabolism, and a special set of enzymes needed for the biosynthesis and metabolic breakdown of the transmitter. Each neuron makes, stores, and releases only one type of transmitter from the many branches of its axonal processes. The special enzymes and other macromolecules needed for the storage and release of a particular transmitter are found only in those neurons using that transmitter. Neurons are thus biochemically differentiated, by virtue of the particular set of transmitter-related macromolecules they contain, into "transmitter-specific" types for the life of the animal. Although the bouton contains all this machinery, and can synthesize and store the transmitter locally, the macromolecules needed to catalyze these processes are synthesized in the cell body or PERIKARYON of the neuron and must be transported down the length of the axon as needed. This may explain why the transmitter and its related enzymes are found throughout the neuron, including the perikaryon and the preterminal axon, although they usually appear in much higher concentrations in the bouton.

The exact mechanism involved in the release of small amounts of transmitter from the presynaptic nerve terminal in response to waves of depolarization associated with the arrival of a nerve impulse at the terminal is not fully understood. The process has been most thoroughly studied at the neuromuscular junction. Here the arrival of a nerve impulse is followed by the release of ACh after a delay of about 0.3-0.4 msec. This burst of released transmitter appears to occur as a consequence of the simultaneous release of the contents of several hundred synaptic vesicles. Shortly after the arrival of the action potential, these vesicles come into temporary contact with the external cell membrane of the nerve terminal, and areas of high permeability are formed in the neuronal membrane through which the vesicle contents are discharged to the exterior, a process known as EXOCYTOSIS. This process seems to be triggered by an inward movement of calcium ions from the extracellular fluid. Transmitter release in this and all other synapses is blocked if calcium is absent from the extracellular fluid. After the vesicles have discharged, they are apparently refilled by local biosynthesis of the transmitter. The presynaptic nerve terminal is always separated from the postsynaptic cell by a gap, the synaptic cleft, containing extracellular fluid. The presynaptic terminal and postsynaptic cell, however, although separate, are tightly held together by fine threads of extracellular protein-mucopolysaccharide. In electron micrographs, the postsynaptic membrane appears thickened at the area of synaptic contact (Fig. 2-6), and sometimes a more complicated postsynaptic "web" structure may be seen. Most importantly, there are specialized receptor molecules in the postsynaptic membrane, which are so placed that the released transmitter diffusing across the cleft interacts with them to initiate the response of the postsynaptic cell. The nature of these receptors is still obscure, but recent studies suggest that they are proteins. Receptor molecules may be membrane proteins, which, in response to the transmitter, open or close pores known as IONOPHORES in the membrane, thus changing the membrane permeability to such inorganic ions as sodium, potassium and chloride. Other types of receptor molecules may act by triggering reactions, catalyzed by membrane-bound enzymes; the end products of these reactions control membrane permeability by other mechanisms. For example, the production of cyclic AMP, which is apparently involved in synaptic transmission by some of the amine transmitters, is transmitter-stimulated.

Although each presynaptic terminal releases only one type of transmitter, the surface of the postsynaptic cell contains many different types of transmitter-receptor sites, since each cell receives inputs from presynaptic terminals using a variety of different transmitters, and receptors are transmitter-specific. It is even quite usual to find more than one type of receptor for a given transmitter; thus ACh interacts with two different types of receptor (see p. 103), which mediate quite different types of post-synaptic responses. Such receptors, however, usually occur on different postsynaptic cells. In skeletal muscle, only one type of cholinergic receptor exists, and these receptors are most dense in those regions of the muscle membrane immediately under the motor nerve terminals (the end-plate region). Whether transmitter receptors are similarly clustered under their appropriate nerve terminals in neurons in the CNS is not known.

Our knowledge of synaptic structure and function allows us to identify the various sites at which drugs may affect synaptic transmission. Drugs can act by altering the properties of (a) the presynaptic terminal and (b) the postsynaptic mechanisms. In the latter category are drugs that act directly on the transmitter receptors as agonists or antagonists of the naturally occurring transmitter. In this case, the "transmitter receptor" and the "drug receptor" are one and the same. There are also numerous sites at which drugs can act on the presynaptic machinery to alter the amount of transmitter released or to prolong its action after release. Some of their possible roles can be listed as follows:

Inhibitors of transmitter biosynthesis. Substances that inhibit one or another of the enzymes responsible for the normal replacement of transmitter in the presynaptic terminal. An alternative mode of action here would be to inhibit the uptake by the terminal of some precursor substance needed for transmitter synthesis.

False transmitters. Substances that are taken up and stored in presynaptic terminals and released in place of the naturally occurring transmitter. Such substances are usually less effective in stimulating the postsynaptic receptors and thus effectively depress synaptic transmission. This group also includes chemicals that can be converted by the normal biosynthetic enzymes into false transmitters.

Inhibitors of transmitter inactivation. Substances that potentiate and prolong the effects of the naturally occurring transmitter by inhibiting the normal mechanisms that terminate these effects at postsynaptic receptor sites. A degradative enzyme [e.g., acetylcholinesterase (AChE)], an "amine pump" mechanism, or both may be involved. For example, in monoaminergic neurons, the degradative enzyme monoamine oxidase (MAO) is present in nerve terminals that use catecholamine transmitters (NE and DA) or 5-HT and regulates the storage level of these amines, but these nerve terminals also possess specific uptake mechanisms that appear to terminate the effects of the amine transmitters. Inhibition of either mechanism tends to potentiate synaptic transmission in such neurons.

Depleting agents. The most widely used agent is the alkaloid, reserpine, which blocks normal storage of NE, DA, and 5-HT in synaptic vesicles and thus leads to a profound and long-lasting depletion of these three amines in the brain and to a block in synaptic transmission in neurons using these transmitters.

Displacing agents. Substances that effect the release of the endogenous transmitter onto receptor sites by displacing it from its neuronal storage sites. Such substances are themselves usually without direct affects on postsynaptic receptors but stimulate these receptors indirectly by releasing the endogenous transmitter.

Because neurons differ from other cells of the body in their biochemical machinery for transmission of nervous impulses, it is not surprising that many neuropharmacological agents act upon this machinery. Drugs that have this type of action are likely to act specifically on neurons, as opposed to other cells. Interference with other aspects of cell metabolism, such as protein synthesis or energy metabolism, is less likely *a priori* to selectively affect nervous system function.

Not all drugs act on the CNS at the synaptic transmission level. Some drugs affect the mechanisms involved in the propagation of nerve impulses in the neuronal membrane. Anesthetic drugs, for example, act to block propagation of the action potentials by changing the properties of the neuronal membrane; other more specific drugs selectively block membrane permeability channels for sodium and potassium, with the same result. The naturally occurring neurotoxins, TETRODOTOXIN (from the Japanese pufferfish) and BATRACHOTOXIN (from the skin of a South American toad), act this way. Such general interference with neuronal function, however, does not affect behavior in ways that can be studied, since such compounds are very toxic. Similarly, such drugs as the cardiac glycosides (e.g., ouabain) that block the active extrusion of sodium from cells and thus lead to depolarization of neurons and other excitable cells, or drugs that interfere with energy metabolism, do not affect behavior in ways that can be readily analyzed, since their action is so diffuse and undirected.

Having outlined some of the ways in which drugs can interact with the nervous system, we will briefly review some of the experimental approaches used by neuropharmacologists to determine how particular drugs work. These are broadly of two types: those measuring the effects of drugs on the electric activity of neurons in the CNS and those studying the effects of drugs by biochemical techniques.

Electrophysiological studies of drug activity in the CNS

Electrophysiology involves the study of electric neuronal activity, using highly sophisticated electronic equipment to amplify, record, and display the extremely small changes in current and voltage associated with such activity. There are two basic approaches: those that measure the over-all electric activity of large populations of neurons and those that measure the electric activity of single neurons.

Neuronal population recording methods

Electroencephalography

This involves the recording of differences in electric potential (in microvolts) between different points on the surface of the

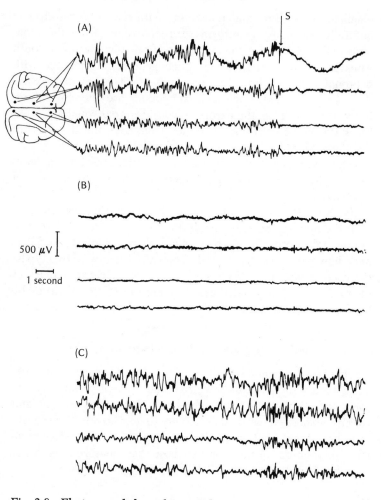

Fig. 2-8 Electroencephalographic records of electric activity in the cerebral cortex of an unanesthetized cat following administration of physostigmine and atropine. (A) Control record with an "arousal response" at S; (B) 10 minutes after 0.08 mg/kg physostigmine sulfate (i.p.); (C) 20 minutes after the subsequent injection of 3 mg/kg atropine sulfate (i.p.). (From Bradley and Elkes, 1957.)

brain; the waves thus obtained are amplified and recorded as an electroencephalogram (EEG). In animals, the relatively large electrodes used are usually placed on the surface of the brain, or inserted into the brain, through openings trephined in the skull; in man, the electrodes are placed on the scalp. Since EEG records are virtually the only form of electric recording feasible in human subjects, the method has been widely used in clinical studies.

Unfortunately, the EEG is a highly complex parameter, since it represents the resultant of electric changes in many thousands of neurons recorded by the electrodes. Nevertheless, the EEG is valuable in providing an over-all index of the state of activation of such areas as the cerebral cortex. Characteristic changes in both the frequency and the amplitude of discharge of the EEG are known to be associated with different states of arousal and attention. Thus, for example, there are EEG changes typical of the various stages of sleep and of arousal, many of which can be mimicked by drugs. Barbiturates tend to produce an EEG pattern similar to that seen in normal slow-wave sleep; amphetamines, on the other hand, induce an EEG pattern characteristic of states of arousal (Fig. 2-8).

Evoked potentials

Evoked potentials are the electric changes, recorded from a relatively large electrode placed extracellularly, when a sensory pathway or remote brain area is stimulated. They represent the net result of complex firing patterns in the population of neurons affected by the stimulus. The pattern of a given evoked potential changes with states of arousal and sleep, and such changes can also be mimicked by certain drugs.

Single cell recording methods

Extracellular recording with electrodes

The activity of single neurons can be monitored in experimental animals by electrodes that usually consist of very fine

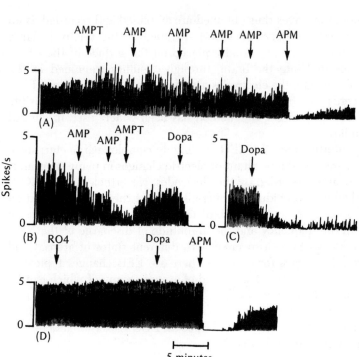

Fig. 2-9 Single cell recordings (rate meter trace) from dopaminergic neurons in the zona compacta of rat substantia nigra. In (A), treatment of animals with α-methyl-p-tyrosine (AMPT) 50 mg/kg prevented amphetamine (AMP) (1.0 mg/kg) inhibition of cell firing. Inhibition of firing by apomorphine (APM) (0.1 mg/kg) is, however, still seen. In (B), α-methyl-p-tyrosine reverses inhibition of cell firing by AMP given before the α-methyl-p-tyrosine. In (C), L-dopa inhibits cell firing similar to that seen after apomorphine. In (D), pretreatment with a large dose of dopa-decarboxylase inhibitor RO 4-4602 (RO4) (800 mg/kg) abolishes the inhibitory effects of L-dopa, although apomorphine inhibition still occurs. These results indicate that the effects of amphetamine and dopa on cell firing are indirect, involving in one case an induced release of endogenous dopamine and in the other conversion of L-dopa. (From Bunney, Aghajanian, and Roth, 1973.)

diameter tungsten wire, insulated so that only the electrode tip records electric activity. By inserting such electrodes into precisely defined brain regions with stereotaxic manipulators, it is possible to record the discharge pattern of single cells in defined anatomical regions of the CNS. It may also be possible to identify the type of neuron from which the recording is being made by stimulating some remote brain region or a neuronal pathway from which the neurons are known to receive input or to which their axons project. For example, pyramidal cells in the cerebral cortex can be identified since they can be made to fire by stimulating the pyramidal tracts, thus evoking a flow of nerve impulses in the axons of these cells back to the cell bodies in the cortex—in the reverse or "antidromic" direction to that in which the impulses normally travel. Figure 2-9 shows the results of an experiment in which amphetamine was found to alter the rate of firing of identified single neurons in the rat substantia nigra.

Extracellular recording with the iontophoretic application of drugs

The use of single cell recording in conjunction with a micromethod for the application of drugs to the immediate vicinity of the cell from which a recording is being made is one of the most powerful techniques of modern neuropharmacology. Application of drugs is by iontophoretic ejection of charged drug molecules from the tip of a finely drawn glass microelectrode. The rate of ejection of the drug can be controlled by regulating the current flowing through the electrode tip. The drug-containing electrode is part of a multi-barreled electrode assembly in which one of the other electrodes is used to monitor the electric activity of the single cell. As many as four to six drug-containing electrodes together with a recording electrode can be used (Fig. 2-10), so that the effects of several drugs on the firing rate of a given cell can be measured. Controls rule out effects due simply to change in pH, passage of electric current, or diffusion of the drug to

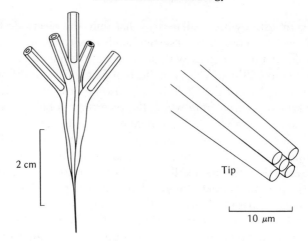

Fig. 2-10 Multi-barreled microelectrode for application of chemicals by micro-electrophoresis.

neighboring neurons. In addition, the amount of drug administered is generally proportional to the iontophoretic current applied through the microelectrode, so that it is possible to construct dose-response curves relating the graded effects of various amounts of drug on neuronal firing (Fig. 2-11). A further refinement introduced in recent years is to study the effects of microiontophoretically applied drugs on physiologically identified neurons, using the methods for identifying single units described above. In this way, far more meaningful data on the pharmacological properties of neuron types in the SNC can be obtained. In much of the older literature, such techniques have not been applied to identified cell populations but simply to randomly selected neurons in a given brain area. Thus it is common to find that out of 100 cells tested with a given drug or transmitter 30% responded by excitation, 35% were inhibited, 25% did not respond at all, and the remaining 10% showed a mixed response with, for example, excitation followed by inhibition. When identified cell

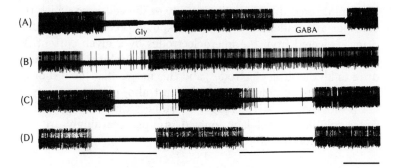

Fig. 2-11   The selective antagonistic action of bicuculline on the response of cuneo-thalamic relay neurons in cat brain to GABA. A continuous film records the firing of a touch cell whose discharge is maintained by constant iontophoretic release of glutamate. Cell responses to glycine and to GABA were tested alternately. The inhibitory responses at 14 na of glycine and GABA in (A) were only just maximal, and bicuculline was released with a current of 168 na, which began approximately 75 seconds before the start of (B) and terminated between (B) and (C), which are continuous with each other and with (D). (Calibration, 5 seconds.) (From Kelly and Renaud, 1973.)

populations are tested, much more consistent results are usually obtained.

Despite the fact that iontophoretic application of drugs is a powerful tool for the direct investigation of drug action on receptor sites in the CNS, the technique has serious drawbacks. The electrode assemblies used are complicated, and the array of electrodes is fairly large. This means that drug application can rarely be restricted to single neurons, especially if they are small (see Fig. 2-10). Furthermore, the insertion of the electrode assembly into the brain necessarily produces some tissue damage in the region from which recordings are to be made. A difficulty in attempting to apply quantitative dose-response analysis to the effects produced by drugs administered iontophoretically is that there is no way of determining precisely what the concentration of administered drug is in the vicinity of the cell from which recordings are made, nor is it always known precisely how much drug is ejected from the microelectrodes by a given current. It is also necessary to use a very concentrated solution of the test drug to fill the drug electrodes, and this means that the test drug must be quite soluble in water; it must also, of course, carry a net positive or negative charge. Substances that are not readily water soluble or that lack ionized groups accordingly are not suitable for iontophoretic application.

Intracellular recording techniques

The action of transmitters or releated drugs on the membrane of postsynaptic cells can be most precisely analyzed when the tip of a very fine recording electrode can be inserted into the cells, while the test substance is iontophoretically administered to the external surface of the cell membrane through an extracellular electrode. This technique has been applied with considerable success to such peripheral synapses as the neuromuscular junction, but it has proved far more difficult to use in the CNS. It has, however, been possible to analyze the action of such CNS transmitters as NE, GABA, and glycine (Gly) in this way. The technique usually involves the construction of an assembly of glass microelectrodes as described above, but with the tip of the recording electrode set slightly in advance of the tips of the drug-containing electrodes. As the electrode assembly is slowly lowered into a brain region, large neurons may be impaled by the tip of the recording electrode, leaving the drug electrodes outside the cell. Because the recording electrode is very easily dislodged from its intracellular position, recording in this way is technically very difficult; a given cell can rarely be recorded from for more than a few seconds. Nevertheless, with such an arrangement, very sophisticated measurements of drug or transmitter action can be made. The test substance can be applied to the external surface of the cell, and changes in membrane potential and membrane resistance can be measured directly via the intracellular electrode.

The biochemical analysis of drug actions on the CNS

In the last decade, biochemical techniques have been applied with increasing frequency and success to the analysis of drug action on neuronal tissue. It is impossible to give more than a survey of the battery of tools now available for such studies and a broad outline of the types of approach possible with them. There are two levels at which biochemical analysis may be made: either by using an isolated preparation of brain slices, homogenates, or individual enzymes, receptor sites, etc., for the *in vitro* analysis of drug effects or by administering a drug to an animal and examining its effect on brain chemistry *in vivo*.

In vitro techniques

The various targets for drug action outlined above (Fig. 2-7) can be isolated or dissected out and examined individually in various *in vitro* systems. For example, a drug that acts as an inhibitor or alternative substrate for enzymes involved in the biosynthesis or breakdown of transmitter substances can be studied directly in a test-tube system of the purified enzyme. Drugs that interfere with other aspects of metabolism, storage, uptake, or release of transmitters in presynaptic nerve terminals can be studied in *in vitro* systems containing presynaptic terminals isolated from brain homogenates. When brain tissue is disrupted by homogenization in an isotonic medium, the presynaptic nerve terminals tend to remain intact as "pinched-off" fragments, which round up to become membrane-bound spherical particles known as SYNAPTOSOMES. The synaptosomes can be harvested from brain homogenates by centrifugation techniques; they represent a useful system for studying drug effects, since they contain the machinery for transmitter metabolism and storage. Since synaptosomes take up and accumulate radioactively labeled transmitters, for example, they can be used to study drugs that inhibit such uptake, which probably represents the normal in-activation process for most transmitters in the CNS. Another widely used *in vitro* preparation is the brain slice. Thin slices of brain tissue remain metabolically viable for several hours if incubated in warm oxygenated saline solution, and they will take up transmitters or their precursors. These slices also re-lease transmitters upon electric stimulation or application of transmitter-displacing drugs. They thus constitute a convenient system for studying the action of drugs on transmitter release processes and various other aspects of presynaptic neurophar-macology.

The analytical methods used for these *in vitro* studies, and for *in vivo* studies of transmitter metabolism, must be very sensitive since the concentration of any one transmitter substance in brain tissue is very low (micrograms per gram wet weight of brain). Such highly sensitive chemical techniques include measuring fluorescence or radioactivity of labeled transmitters or precursors.

A recent breakthrough in *in vitro* studies has been the devel-opment of methods that allow postsynaptic receptor mechanisms to be studied biochemically. One approach involves the use of some antagonist or agonist drug that binds with a very high affinity and specificity to receptor sites. The drug is radioactively labeled, and its binding to intact tissues, to membrane fractions isolated from homogenates, or even to solubilized membrane proteins can be used to identify and quantify the receptor sites present. For example, the snake venom, α-BUNGAROTOXIN, binds with high specificity and affinity to cholinergic receptor sites on the surface of skeletal muscle—where it is a powerful antagonist —so that it can be used as a label to identify, count, and aid in the further isolation and purification of these receptor molecules. The binding of a labeled antagonist drug to membrane fractions that can be blocked by simultaneous incubation with non-radio-active agonists or antagonists of a given receptor can also be used as a biochemical index to identify and quantify drug and transmitter receptor sites in homogenates or slices of the mammalian CNS. Receptors for morphine and related opiate drugs and for Gly and ACh have recently been studied this way.

In vivo techniques

One often-used approach has been to administer a drug to an animal and measure the changes in the concentration of transmitters or other chemical components of the brain. This technique was used to show that the alkaloid, reserpine, caused a profound and long-lasting depletion of catecholamines and 5-HT in the CNS. Changes in the steady-state concentration of chemical constituents of the cell in response to drug treatments, however, afford less information than dynamic changes induced by drugs during release, resynthesis, or breakdown of the constituent being studied. Drugs may affect the rate of metabolic turnover of transmitters without necessarily changing the steady-state level. Transmitter turnover can be estimated by using a radioactively labeled transmitter or transmitter precursor and following the rate of appearance and disappearance of the labeled material in the brain. An index of the rate of turnover can sometimes also be obtained by measuring the concentration of transmitter metabolites present in the brain, since a more rapid breakdown of a transmitter (implying faster release and utilization in neuronal pathways) often leads to an accumulation of one or other of its degradative products. Homovanillic acid, for example, is the major metabolite formed during the breakdown of DA in the brain. The concentration of this metabolite is increased under conditions in which DA release is accelerated, as is found after the administration of drugs that antagonize DA at its receptor sites in the CNS. Such receptor blockade causes a reflex increase in the rate of firing of dopaminergic neurons, which is interpreted as an attempt to counteract the effect of the drug. This is seen biochemically as an increase in DA turnover and an accumulation of homovanillic acid. By such tortuous reasoning are experiments in neurochemical pharmacology devised! The concept of "receptor feedback," as exemplified above, is useful in the analysis of agonist and antagonist drugs in the CNS, since antagonists generally increase the turnover of the transmitter whose receptors are blocked, whereas agonists tend to have the converse effect, selectively slowing turnover of the transmitter in question.

Other techniques are available that allow direct measurements of transmitter release to be made in intact brain preparations, although these usually involve the use of a fully anesthetized animal. Cannulae can be implanted into the CSF to perfuse the ventricular system or into the brain itself to perfuse a local region. Transmitter release can also be measured on the surface of the brain by means of a saline-filled collection cup placed there. The minute amounts of transmitter collected in such experiments often makes it necessary to prelabel the brain transmitter stores with radioactive transmitter or precursor in order to detect the material released. The effects of drugs on transmitter release evoked by electric or reflex stimulation of remote pathways or drug-induced release can then be studied. In recent years, techniques have been devised that allow such collection experiments to be performed on conscious animals by means of chronically implanted cannulae, thus permitting such studies to be undertaken during normal behavior.

Neuropharmacology of individual neurotransmitter systems

Acetylcholine

Drug effects on metabolism (for review see Marchbanks, 1975)

Acetylcholine (ACh) is synthesized from choline and the acetyl donor substance acetyl coenzyme A (acetyl-CoA) in cholinergic nerve terminals; this reaction is catalyzed by the enzyme CHOLINE ACETYL TRANSFERASE (ChAc). Acetyl-CoA is formed during the metabolism of carbohydrates and fats in all living cells, but the choline needed for ACh synthesis depends upon a special membrane transport mechanism present only in cholinergic neurons. This uptake system has a very high affinity for choline and operates efficiently at external choline concentrations as low as 1 μM (Yamamura and Snyder, 1973). A low-affinity choline uptake that operates at much higher concentrations (100 μM) is present in many cells that use choline for the biosynthesis of phospholipids. In the CNS, the biosynthetic enzyme ChAc is found only in cholinergic neurons; it is found in abundance in synaptosome fractions isolated from brain homogenates, which contain as much as 80% of the total tissue activity, indicating that most of the enzyme is localized in pre-synaptic nerve terminals. The biosynthesis of transmitter takes place in the cytoplasm of cholinergic terminals, but the resulting ACh is stored mainly within the synaptic vesicles in this cyto-plasm. No drugs are known that act as specific inhibitors of ChAc, but one potent inhibitor of ACh synthesis is known. This is the compound HEMICHOLINIUM (HC3) (Fig. 2-12), which acts as a powerful inhibitor of the high affinity choline uptake system in the neuronal membrane, thus blocking the entry into the neuron of a vital precursor that cannot be synthesized locally within the cholinergic neuron. Unfortunately, HC3 does not penetrate readily into the CNS after systemic administration, al-though some penetration has been obtained by direct applica-tion on the brain or into the CSF.

Acetylcholine is metabolically degraded within cholinergic nerve terminals, and after its release from such terminals, by the enzyme ACETYLCHOLINESTERASE (AChE), which hydrolyzes the transmitter to acetate and choline. The enzyme is present in or attached to the cellular and intracellular membranes of the pre-synaptic cholinergic neurons, but it is also present on the mem-brane of the postsynaptic or "cholinoceptive" cell. Acetylcho-linesterase is an unusual enzyme in having an extremely high rate of catalytic action, a single molecule of enzyme being able to catalyze the breakdown of more than 100,000 molecules of

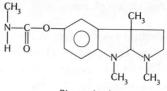

Physostigmine

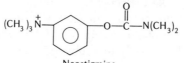

Neostigmine

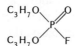

Diisopropylfluorophosphonate

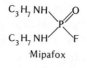

Mipafox

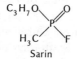

Sarin

(A) Inhibitors of Acetylcholinesterase

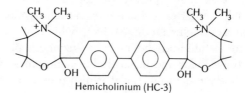

Hemicholinium (HC-3)

(B) Inhibitors of acetylcholine biosynthesis

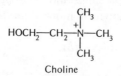

Choline

(C) Choline-precursor for acetylcholine biosynthesis

ACh per minute. It is thus ideally suited for its main task, which is to inactivate ACh after release from cholinergic nerve terminals. This inactivation is by conversion of the transmitter to pharmacologically inert metabolites; since the enzyme is situated on the post- and presynaptic membranes, it has ready access to ACh in the synaptic cleft. In addition, AChE regulates the storage level of transmitter within the presynatic terminal by degrading any ACh synthesized in excess of the storage capacity of the synaptic vesicles. Numerous drugs are available that act as selective and potent inhibitors of AChE (Fig. 2-12). Not all of these compounds, however, penetrate into the CNS after systemic administration. PHYSOSTIGMINE and such organophosphorus inhibitors as DIISOPROPYLFLUOROPHOSPHONATE (DFP) and SARIN have high CNS activity, whereas NEOSTIGMINE has little or no CNS activity owing to its poor penetration of the blood-brain barrier.

Few drugs are known that affect ACh storage or release. BOTULINUM TOXINS act specifically to block the release of ACh normally evoked by nerve impulses from cholinergic terminals, but they have little or no CNS application.

Agonist and antagonist drugs at cholinergic receptors

Although there are relatively few drugs that affect presynaptic cholinergic mechanisms, many drugs act as agonists or antagonists at postsynaptic cholinergic receptors. Two major categories of cholinergic receptor site are known, the MUSCARINIC and the NICOTINIC. In the peripheral nervous system, muscarinic receptors are found in all the postsynaptic cells innervated by the parasympathetic nervous system; the action of the vagus nerve in slowing the heart, for example, is mediated by such receptors. These are identified by the use of the drug MUSCARINE (Fig. 2-13), which mimics the actions of ACh on such receptor sites. Other agonists that are selective for muscarinic sites are ACETYL-

---

Fig. 2-12 Drugs that act on the synthesis and breakdown of acetylcholine.

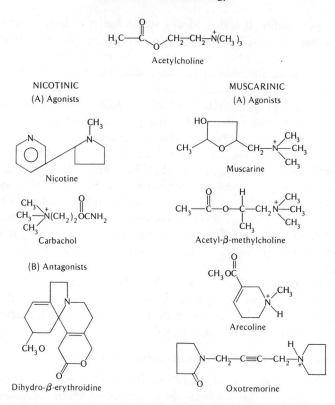

Fig. 2-13 Agonists and antagonists at cholinergic synapses.

β-METHYLCHOLINE, ARECOLINE, PILOCARPINE, and OXOTREMORINE. The latter substance has high CNS activity; as its name implies, it induces a Parkinson-like tremor in experimental animals. Acetylcholine itself and acetyl-β-methylcholine and arecoline penetrate only very poorly into the CNS after systemic administration.

ATROPINE is the classical muscarine antagonist drug, and several related substances, such as HYOSCINE (SCOPOLAMINE) and BENZTROPINE, have similar effects; all three drugs act centrally.

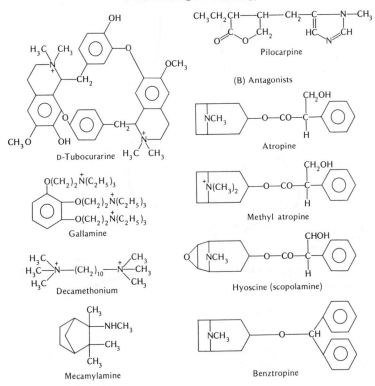

Pilocarpine

(B) Antagonists

Atropine

Methyl atropine

Hyoscine (scopolamine)

Benztropine

D-Tubocurarine

Gallamine

Decamethonium

Mecamylamine

METHYL ATROPINE is a useful tool, since it is a potent antagonist peripherally but does not penetrate the blood-brain barrier to any significant extent. By comparing the effects of systemically applied atropine and methyl atropine, it is thus possible to assess whether an observed effect is due to central or peripheral anticholinergic drug activity.

The nicotinic category of cholinergic receptor is so named because the action of ACh on such sites is mimicked by the drug NICOTINE. Two subcategories of nicotinic receptor exist in the peripheral nervous system, one on skeletal muscles mediating the effects of ACh on neuromuscular junctions, the other mediating the effects of ACh on autonomic ganglia. These two sub-

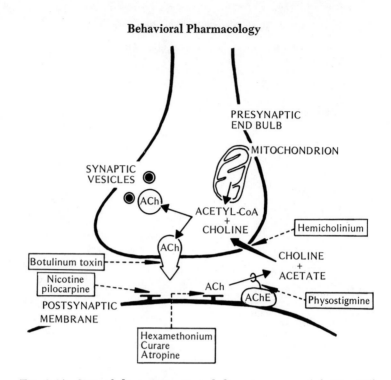

Fig. 2-14   Sites of drug action at a cholinergic synapse (cf. Fig. 2-7). (From Rech and Moore, 1971.)

categories differ slightly in their sensitivity to drugs, and particularly to antagonists. All nicotonic receptors are selectively stimulated by the agonist drugs NICOTINE and CARBAMYLCHOLINE (CARBACHOL) (Fig. 2-14). The antagonists D-TUBOCURARINE, GALLAMINE, and DECAMETHONIUM act primarily on nicotinic receptors in muscle, whereas HEXAMETHONIUM, MECAMYLAMINE, PEMPIDINE, and CHLORISONDAMINE are selective ganglion-blocking drugs. None of these drugs penetrate the blood-brain barrier to any significant extent, although they can be used centrally if injected directly into the CSF or the brain.

In studying the molecular basis of both nicotinic and muscarinic receptor action, the use of α-bungarotoxin has allowed progress to be made in isolating and purifying nicotinic receptors from skeletal muscle and from the electric organs of electric eels and fish; these latter are excellent sources for such receptors. The muscarinic actions of ACh in such peripheral organs as the heart, and possibly also the brain, have been found to be associated with increased production of the cyclic nucleotide cyclic-3'5'-guanosine monophosphate (cyclic GMP), suggesting that stimulation of muscarinic receptors by ACh leads to a stimulation of guanyl cyclase, the enzyme responsible for synthesis of this nucleotide. How cyclic GMP then affects cell permeability to produce the characteristic tissue responses elicited by muscarinic stimulation is not yet known.

Cholinergic receptors in the CNS

The iontophoretic application of ACh evokes a response in a varying proportion of neurons in different brain regions. The response is usually excitatory, although some cells show only depression of firing and some may show excitation followed by depression. There are only a few clearly defined systems in which cholinergic responses of known cell types have been analyzed. One of these is the Renshaw cell in the spinal cord. These cells are small inhibitory interneurons situated near large motor neurons in the ventral horn; they receive a cholinergic excitatory input from collateral axon branches of the cholinergic motor nerves as they leave the spinal cord. The Renshaw cells, in turn, send an inhibitory input to the motor neurons, thus constituting a self-damping feedback loop for motor neuron activity. The effects of ACh on Renshaw cells have been extensively studied; the cells can be easily identified, since they are excited when motor nerves are stimulated antidromically. Iontophoretically applied ACh mimics the normal excitatory synaptic potentials of these cells; ACh activity appears to be mediated mainly by nicotinic receptors, i.e., the effects are mimicked by nicotine and carbachol and blocked by dihydro-β-erythroidine and d-tubocurarine, whereas atropine blocks the effects only weakly.

In contrast, cholinergic responses in most supraspinal regions of the CNS, such as the hypothalamus, basal ganglia, and cerebral cortex, appear to be predominantly muscarinic in character. The action of ACh iontophoretically applied to physiologically identified pyramidal Betz cells in the cortex has been especially thorougly studied. A high proportion of these cells are excited by iontophoretically applied ACh; muscarine rather than nicotine mimics this action, and atropine rather than dihydro-β-erythroidine blocks it. It is thus clear that receptors with properties similar to nicotinic and muscarinic sites in the periphery exist in the CNS, although it is difficult to say whether the CNS receptors have identical properties to those in the periphery because of the difficulty of obtaining precise quantitative data on the potencies of nicotinic and muscarinic agonists and antagonists in the CNS.

Catecholamines (for reviews see Iversen, 1967; Iversen, 1973; Usdin and Snyder, 1974)

The catecholamines DA and NE are present in specific neuronal pathways in the mammalian CNS, where they almost certainly act as transmitters. Epinephrine is formed from norepinephrine but is present in mammals mainly as an adrenal medullary hormone, occurring only in trace amounts in the CNS. Although DA and NE are present in different neuronal pathways in the CNS, and serve independent transmitter functions, the basic pharmacological and biochemical properties of the two types of adrenergic neuron are so similar that the effects of drugs on the presynaptic adrenergic terminals will not be considered separately.

Drug effects on metabolism

The catecholamines are synthesized from the amino acids L-phenylalanine and L-tyrosine by a multi-enzyme pathway in

Fig. 2-15 Synthesis and metabolism of the catecholamines. MAO, monoamine oxidase; COMT, catechol-O-methyl transferase.

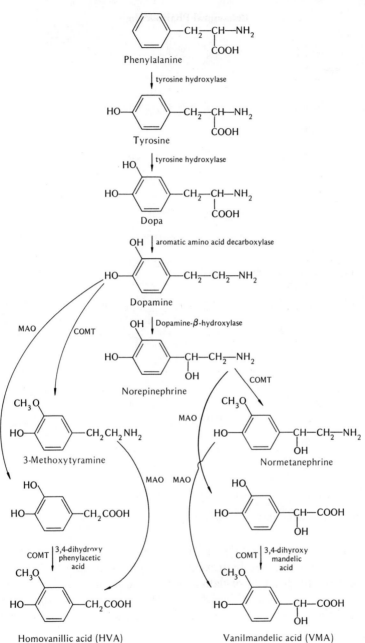

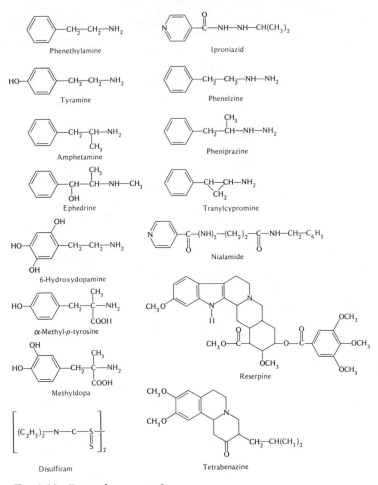

Fig. 2-16   Drugs that act at adrenergic synapses.

adrenergic neurons (Fig. 2-15). The enzyme TYROSINE HYDROX-YLASE catalyzes the hydroxylation of phenylalanine to tyrosine and the further hydroxylation of tyrosine to the catechol amino acid L-dopa. This is decarboxylated by AROMATIC AMINO ACID DECARBOXYLASE (sometimes called DOPA-DECARBOXYLASE), and the produced DA is converted to NE by another hydroxylating enzyme DOPAMINE-β-HYDROXYLASE. Dopaminergic neurons lack the latter enzyme, and DA is thus the end product of biosynthesis in these cells. The other two enzymes are present in both types of adrenergic neuron, and, in each case, tyrosine hydroxylase has a much lower activity than aromatic amino acid decarboxylase, thus catalyzing the slowest step in the pathway and governing the over-all rate of catecholamine synthesis. The tyrosine hydroxylase reaction is regulated by the concentration of end product (DA or NE) present in the presynaptic nerve terminals, since the enzyme is inhibited by high concentrations of these amines. This constitutes a negative feedback control system, which adjusts the rate of catecholamine synthesis to meet the moment to moment demands for transmitter release. Tyrosine hydroxylase and aromatic amino acid decarboxylase are present in the cytoplasm of the adrenergic nerve terminals, whereas dopamine-β-hydroxylase is strictly localized to the membranes of synaptic vesicles in noradrenergic terminals. Since tyrosine hydroxylase is the rate-limiting enzyme for the over-all pathway, drugs that inhibit this enzyme are the most effective in limiting the over-all rate of catecholamine biosynthesis. The most commonly used inhibitor of tyrosine hydroxylase is the amino acid α-METHYL-p-TYROSINE (Fig. 2-16), which is an effective inhibitor of the enzyme *in vitro* and *in vivo*. After administration *in vivo*, this compound causes a near total inhibition of DA and NE synthesis in all parts of the body, which lasts for 6 to 8 hours. Because α-methyltyrosine is not very soluble, the methyl ester, which is more soluble in water, is often used for *in vivo* administration; this compound is converted to α-methyltyrosine in the body. Other inhibitors of tyrosine hydroxylase that are effective *in vivo* are 3-IODOTYROSINE and 3-IODO-α-METHYLTYROSINE, but their effects are of shorter duration and less specific than the effects of α-methyltyrosine, since the iodotyrosines are also involved in the metabolism of the thyroid hormone thyroxin.

It is possible to inhibit the synthesis of NE without affecting that of DA by using drugs that act as inhibitors of dopamine-β-hydroxylase; these include DISULFIRAM (DIETHYLDITHIOCARBA-MATE) and FLA-63 (Fig. 2-16). Although these compounds are effective inhibitors of NE synthesis *in vivo*, they are, unfortunately, not very specific, since they both act by forming complexes with copper, which is present as an integral part of the enzyme dopamine-β-hydroxylase. These drugs thus tend to inhibit a variety of other copper-dependent enzymes and are more toxic and less specific than one would wish, for drugs that are used in behavioral studies.

Another way in which drugs can interact with the catecholamine biosynthetic pathway is as substrates for one or another of the enzymes involved. Thus, L-DOPA is a useful substance for systemic administration, since, unlike the catecholamines, it penetrates the blood-brain barrier and is converted in the CNS to DA and, to a lesser extent, NE. A related amino acid, 3,4-DIHY-DROXYPHENYLSERINE (DOPS), also enters the CNS and is converted by decarboxylation directly to NE. The NE formed after DOPS administration may not necessarily be in appropriate cellular locations, however, since the amino acid can be decarboxylated by aromatic amino acid decarboxylase in DA and 5-HT neurons as well as in noradrenergic neurons. The amino acids α-METHYL-DOPA and α-METHYL-METATYROSINE also enter the brain and can be metabolized to the amines α-methyltyramine, metaraminol, α-methyldopamine, and α-methylnorepinephrine. These amines can be stored and released from adrenergic neurons, and their effects are generally less potent than those of the normal catecholamines; they thus act as "false transmitters," diluting and diminishing the effectiveness of the naturally occurring transmitters.

Metabolically, NE and DA are degraded by similar pathways involving two enzymes: catechol-O-methyltransferase (COMT) and monoamine oxidase (MAO) (Fig. 2-15). These two enzymes, unlike AChE, are not localized at adrenergic synapses, but are widely distributed in neurons and glial cells of the CNS and peripheral tissue. Both enzymes, however, are present in adrenergic neurons, with COMT localized in the cytoplasm and MAO in the mitochondria. The latter enzyme in particular seems to play an important role in regulating the steady-state storage level of NE and DA in adrenergic neurons. Inhibitors of COMT include the simple aromatic compounds CATECHOL and PYRO-GALLOL and the more potent ISOPROPYLTROPOLONE (THUJAPLICIN). Numerous inhibitors of MAO are known, and many of these compounds are used clinically in the treatment of depression (Fig. 2-16); they include such hydrazine analogues of the catecholamines as IPRONIAZID, PHENELZINE, and PHENIPRAZINE and such non-hydrazines as PARGYLINE and TRANYLCYPROMINE. All of these compounds can produce a marked and long-lasting inhibition of MAO *in vivo*, the effects of a single dose persisting for several days. After administration of an MAO inhibitor, the concentrations of DA and NE in the CNS and peripheral tissues are increased, often by more than 100% over normal steady-state concentrations. Neither COMT nor MAO are specific for the catecholamines; COMT will catalyze the methylation of a variety of substrates that have a catechol grouping in the molecule, and MAO will oxidatively deaminate many different amines. Substrates for MAO include the indolamine transmitter 5-HT (see p. 122) and various phenylethylamine and indolamine drugs related in structure to the catecholamines or to 5-HT. Drugs that have an α-methyl substituent adjacent to the amine group, however, are not substrates for MAO. Thus, the false transmitter amines α-methyldopamine and α-methylnorepinephrine are not degraded by MAO, and this is one factor contributing to the persistence of these substances in adrenergic neurons after administration of their precursors.

Drug effects on other aspects of presynaptic adrenergic mechanisms

There are various other sites of drug activity at adrenergic terminals (cf. Fig. 2-7). The catecholamines are inactivated after their release mainly by processes of re-uptake, whereby released amines are taken up from the extracellular fluid by high-affinity transport systems located in the axonal membrane of the pre-synaptic terminals. The uptake systems in dopaminergic and noradrenergic neurons in the CNS are similar in their basic properties, but they differ in their sensitivity to drug inhibition. Thus, although some substances such as AMPHETAMINE and COCAINE, act as potent inhibitors of both systems, other drugs are more potent inhibitors of one rather than the other. The most striking difference in drug sensitivity is the effects of such tricyclic antidepressants as IMIPRAMINE and AMITRIPTYLINE, and their derivatives. These substances are very potent inhibitors of the uptake system in NE-containing neurons, acting at concentrations as low as 0.01 μM, but they are one hundred to one thousand times less potent as inhibitors of the DA uptake system in dopaminergic nerve terminals. Conversely, some drugs, notably the anti-parkinsonian drug BENZTROPINE (Fig. 2-13), are more potent inhibitors of DA than of NE uptake; benztropine is approximately thirty times more effective in the former system. Benztropine has already been described as an anticholinergic drug of the atropine type; its potent effects on DA uptake sites illustrates the common finding that drugs may have multiple sites of action in CNS tissues—a fact that always makes interpretation of drug effects on behavior in neuropharmacological terms extremely difficult. Hardly any drugs have completely specific, single neuropharmacological sites of action, and yet we must argue from the known pharmacological effects of drugs to interpret their mode of action in eliciting behavioral changes. One partial solution to this problem is to test many drugs on a given system. If a given behavioral syndrome is always associated with drugs having a particular neuropharmacological site of action, a more convincing case for the existence of a causal relationship between these phenomena may be established, since other secondary pharmacological activities of a group of drugs are unlikely to be similar.

The storage of catecholamines at adrenergic nerve terminals involves complex chemical mechanisms within the synaptic vesicles, whereby very high concentrations of catecholamine are maintained inside these vesicles by the formation of a complex with the nucleotide adenosine triphosphate (ATP). These storage mechanisms also represent a target for drug action. The alkaloid RESERPINE (Fig. 2-16) and some of its derivatives and TETRABENAZINE and its derivatives act to block the vesicle amine storage system; these drugs can severely deplete catecholamines and 5-HT in adrenergic neurons in the brain and peripheral nervous system. The amine is released from its normal storage sites and degraded by MAO within the adrenergic terminals, and no massive release of catecholamine outside the nerve terminal occurs after reserpine administration; the resulting depletion is very long lasting. It may take 1 or 2 weeks for the CNS concentrations of DA and NE to return to normal. Tetrabenazine has a similar mode of action, but its effects are of much shorter duration, with amine concentrations returning to normal within 24 hours. Another important group of drugs also affect catecholamine storage sites, but they act by displacing the catecholamines and promoting their release into the extracellular fluid, thus mimicking the effects normally produced by adrenergic nerve activity. These compounds are all structural analogues of NE and DA and belong to a large group of phenylethylamine compounds that have pharmacological activity similar to that of the catecholamines; they are known as the SYMPATHOMIMETIC AMINES. Drugs that mimic catecholamine actions by displacing NE and DA from their normal storage sites are termed "indirectly" acting sympathomimetics, in contrast to directly acting sympathomimetics that mimic amine actions by functioning as agonists at adrenergic receptor sites on postsynaptic tissues (see below). Some of the sympathomimetic amines may show both types of activity, acting directly as an agonist and also displacing catecholamines from adrenergic terminals. The activity of such purely indirectly acting sympathomimetics as PHENYLETHYLAMINE, OCTOPAMINE, TYRAMINE, and AMPHETAMINE is easily distinguished, since their sympathomimetic effects disappear when the adrenergic terminals are destroyed surgically or by chemical sympathectomy or when catecholamine stores are depleted with reserpine or by the synthesis inhibitor α-methyl-p-tyrosine.

Certain drugs affect adrenergic nerve terminals because they are substrates for the amine uptake mechanisms; they are thus selectively concentrated within adrenergic neurons as opposed to other tissues of the body. One group of substances known as ADRENERGIC NEURON BLOCKING DRUGS, such as BRETYLIUM and GUANETHIDINE, act in this way to block the normal release of catecholamines from sympathetic nerves in response to nerve stimulation. These drugs are selectively taken up by adrenergic nerve terminals, where they act in a manner like that of local anesthetics to block the transmission of nerve impulses in the fine adrenergic nerve terminals. The adrenergic neuron-blocking drugs, however, do not penetrate the blood-brain barrier and do not act on the CNS. Another compound that is selectively concentrated by adrenergic nerves has a more dramatic effect. The compound 6-HYDROXYDOPAMINE (Fig. 2-16) is taken up by adrenergic nerve terminals; there it reacts to produce a permanent degeneration. 6-Hydroxydopamine acts on both dopaminergic and noradrenergic neurons in the CNS, provided it is directly introduced into the brain or CSF, and it can cause a permanent and near total loss of the catecholamine nerve terminals in the brain and spinal cord in experimental animals. It has proved a most useful research tool for investigating the activity of drugs thought to exert effects via the above pathways.

Agonists and antagonists at adrenergic receptors

As is the case for ACh, the actions of NE in the peripheral sympathetic nervous system are mediated by two categories of postsynaptic receptor site, the α- and β-ADRENOCEPTORS. α-Adrenoceptors mediate the action of NE in causing contraction of vascular smooth muscle cells and are thus important in controlling blood pressure by regulating peripheral resistance. β-Adrenoceptors mediate the action of NE in stimulating the contraction of heart muscle or in causing relaxation of smooth muscle cells in the intestine and bronchi. These two types of receptor are thus not simply excitatory or inhibitory, but are distinguished rather by the fact that they have different agonist and antagonist specificities, as are nicotinic and muscarinic cholinergic receptors. Both types of receptor respond to the catecholamines norepinephrine, epinephrine (E), and ISOPRO-TERENOL, but the order of potencies of these agonists on the two receptors is quite different, being, for α-adrenoceptors, NE = E> ISOPR and, for β-adrenoceptors, ISOPR> E = NE. There are also different antagonist drugs that selectively block one or the other of the receptor types (Fig. 2-17). Among the α-adrenoceptor antagonists are PHENOXYBENZAMINE, DIBENAMINE, PHENTOLAMINE, TOLAZOLINE, and YOHIMBINE, all of which can act centrally. β-Adrenoceptor antagonists include DICHLOROISOPRENALINE, BUTOXAMINE, and PROPRANOLOL.

There is little convincing evidence that dopaminergic neurons exist outside the CNS in mammals, so the pharmacology of DA receptor sites is far less clearly understood than that of NE receptor sites, which have been studied mainly in peripheral tissue preparations. Recent studies of DA receptor sites in the CNS, however, suggest that APOMORPHINE and related derivatives and PIRIBEDIL (ET495) can act as more or less selective agonists, whereas antagonists of a more or less selective nature include the neuroleptic drugs CHLORPROMAZINE and related PHENOTHIAZINES, HALOPERIDOL and related BUTYROPHENONES, PIMOZIDE, and CLOZAPINE (Figs. 4-18, 4-19). Some of these drugs, notably chlorpromazine, are also quite potent antagonists at α-adrenoceptors, and, in addition, have other properties as local anesthetics. Nevertheless, an overlapping specificity between dopaminergic and noradrenergic receptor sites might be expected in view of the close structural similarity between DA and NE. There is suffi-

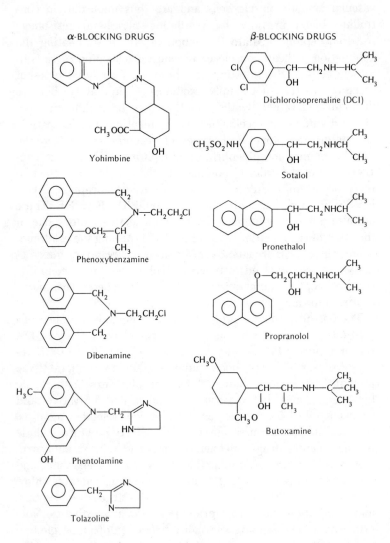

Fig. 2-17 Antagonists at adrenergic receptors.

cient evidence that the receptor sites for DA do belong to a separate category that is distinguishable from either α- or β-adrenoceptors.

Adrenergic receptors in the CNS

There is not sufficient evidence to state that the effect of NE on CNS neurons is due to an interaction with α- and β-adrenoceptors as in the periphery. Although iontophoretically applied NE consistently evokes inhibitory responses in many neurons to which it is applied, there is also evidence that excitatory responses can be evoked in some neurons. The proportion of cells in a given brain area that are excited by NE, however, is sensitive to various features of the experimental design, such as the anesthetic employed and the pH of the iontophoretic solution. It has even been argued that excitatory responses may be artifacts, which occur only as a secondary response to the local vasoconstriction of cerebral blood vessels caused by the diffusion of NE from the site of its application. Such vasoconstriction could, in turn, lead to a local hypoxia to cause neuronal excitation. This would be consistent with reports that excitatory responses to NE are blocked by α-adrenoceptor antagonist drugs. Yet other evidence suggests that cerebral blood vessels do not respond by vasoconstriction to applied NE, so the situation remains confused. Inhibitory responses to NE, however, are well documented in many brain regions and may represent the predominant action of NE on neurons in the CNS. Such responses are blocked by β-adrenoceptor antagonists, indicating that they are similar to β-adrenoceptor responses in the periphery. A further point of similarity is the observation that in both the periphery and the CNS β-adrenoceptor responses to NE appear to involve stimulation of an adenylate cyclase, leading to the increased production of cyclic AMP. In the cerebellum, the inhibitory responses of Purkinje cells to applied NE can be mimicked by iontophoretically applied cyclic AMP, and responses to both cyclic AMP and NE are enhanced by inhibitors of phosphodiesterase, which normally breaks down cyclic AMP (THEOPHYLLINE, PAPAVERINE). Furthermore, the responses are blocked by PROSTAGLANDIN E1, as in the periphery. But inhibitory responses in other brain regions, such as the cerebral cortex, do not necessarily involve the adenylate cyclase-cyclic AMP system, since cyclic AMP does not appear to mimic NE in such regions.

As stated above, receptors for dopamine exist in regions of the CNS that have a preponderance of dopamine-containing nerve terminals, and these differ from both α- and β-adrenoceptors in their pharmacological properties.

5-HT (for review see Green and Grahame-Smith, 1975)

5-HT-Containing neurons exist in the CNS and probably also in the intestine. We know far less about the properties and pharmacology of such neuronal systems, however, than we do about ACh and the catecholamines, probably because 5-HT has not been clearly established as a neurotransmitter at any peripheral synapse.

Drug actions on metabolism and other presynaptic mechanisms

5-HT is synthesized from the plasma amino acid L-tryptophan in a two-step pathway involving hydroxylation by TRYPTOPHAN HYDROXYLASE and decarboxylation of the product (L-5-hydroxytryptophan) by AROMATIC AMINO ACID DECARBOXYLASE (Fig. 2-18). It appears that the latter enzyme is the same as that responsible for decarboxylating L-dopa in adrenergic neurons. Tryptophan hydroxylase is susceptible to inhibition by the amino acid L-*p* CHLOROPHENYLALANINE (PCPA), and this is one of the effective inhibitors of 5-HT biosynthesis available for *in vivo* studies. A single dose of PCPA can inhibit 5-HT synthesis for many hours. The rate of 5-HT biosynthesis is sensitive to the availability of L-tryptophan in blood and brain, since the normal con-

---

Fig. 2-18 Synthesis and metabolism of 5-hydroxytryptamine (5-HT) and some drugs that affect tryptaminergic mechanisms.

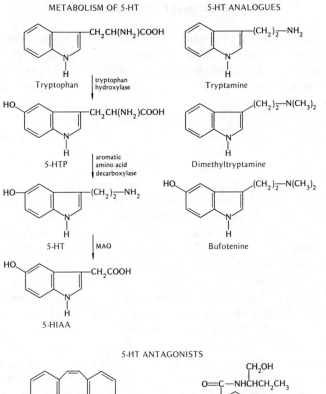

METABOLISM OF 5-HT

Tryptophan

tryptophan hydroxylase

5-HTP

aromatic amino acid decarboxylase

5-HT

MAO

5-HIAA

5-HT ANALOGUES

Tryptamine

Dimethyltryptamine

Bufotenine

5-HT ANTAGONISTS

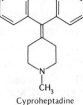

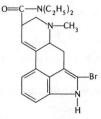

Cyproheptadine

Methysergide '

2-Bromlysergic acid diethylamide

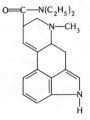

Lysergic acid diethylamide

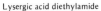

centration of the precursor amino acid seems to be below the threshold for saturation of the biosynthetic enzyme tryptophan hydroxylase. In catecholamine biosynthesis, on the other hand, the concentration of L-tyrosine is less important, since normal tissue concentrations are well above the saturation point for tyrosine hydroxylase. 5-HT synthesis in the CNS can thus be increased by the administration of the precursor L-TRYPTOPHAN and inhibited by the administration of amino acids, such as LEUCINE and VALINE, that compete with tryptophan for transport into the brain from plasma. 5-HT synthesis in the CNS can also be stimulated by the administration of L-5-hydroxytryptophan, which, like L-dopa, penetrates the blood-brain barrier.

5-HT is degraded metabolically by MAO, which is also found in adrenergic neurons. This appears to be the only important metabolic route for 5-HT breakdown in the CNS, leading to the formation of the metabolite 5-HYDROXYINDOLEACETIC ACID (5-HIAA) (Fig. 2-18). All the inhibitors of MAO described above are also effective in preventing 5-HT breakdown in the brain. Like the catecholamines, however, free extracellular 5-HT appears to be removed not by metabolic breakdown but by a re-uptake mechanism located in the membranes of 5-HT-containing nerve terminals. This uptake system is a high-affinity mechanism with a high specificity for 5-HT. It is inhibited by various indolamine analogues of 5-HT, such as TRYPTAMINE, α-METHYL-TRYPTAMINE, and α-METHYL-5-HT. 5-HT uptake is also inhibited by many of the tricyclic antidepressants drugs, which act as potent inhibitors of NE uptake sites. But the exact structure-activity relationships for inhibition of 5-HT and NE uptake by these compounds are not the same. For example, NE uptake sites are inhibited by the imipramine analogues DESIPRAMINE and 3-CHLOROIMIPRAMINE, but the order of potency is desipramine > imipramine > chloroimipramine, whereas the order of potency of these drugs as inhibitors of 5-HT uptake is reversed, chloro-imipramine being the most potent inhibitor.

5-HT storage sites in tryptaminergic neurons are sensitive to

RESERPINE and related drugs, as are the sites in adrenergic neurons, another point of similarity between the 5-HT- and catecholamine-containing structures.

Drug actions on 5-HT receptors (see Aghajanian, 1974)

Receptors for 5-HT have not been well defined, even in peripheral smooth muscle, such as that from the intestine and uterus, which responds to the amine. In the intestine, two types of 5-HT receptor appear to be present: one is antagonized by LYSERGIC ACID derivatives, METHYSERGIDE, and CYPROHEPTADINE (Fig. 2-18), and the other is antagonized by MORPHINE. Whether either or both of these types of receptor exist in the CNS, however, is still uncertain. Responses of neurons to iontophoretically applied 5-HT are usually inhibitory, and such responses have only occasionally been found to be blocked by lysergic acid. It is also not clear what the agonist specificity of CNS receptor sites for 5-HT is. A number of structurally related indolamines, notably N-DIMETHYLTRYPTAMINE, PSILOCIN, and BUFOTENIN (Fig. 2-18), are powerful hallucinogens; it is tempting to speculate that these drugs interact with 5-HT receptors, but this remains to be established.

GABA, glycine, and glutamic acid (Fig. 2-19)

If little is known about the neuropharmacology of indolamine systems in CNS, even less is known about the properties of the neuronal systems that use these amino acid transmitters. GABA is now generally recognized to be the most important inhibitory transmitter in the mammalian CNS. It is found in all regions of the brain and spinal cord and probably is the transmitter in as many as one-third of all synaptic terminals in the brain. Glycine has a more circumscribed function, since its inhibitory transmitter role is restricted to the spinal cord, the lower brain stem, and, possibly, the retina. Glutamic acid is not yet firmly established as a transmitter, but it seems likely that it is a major excitatory transmitter in the mammalian CNS.

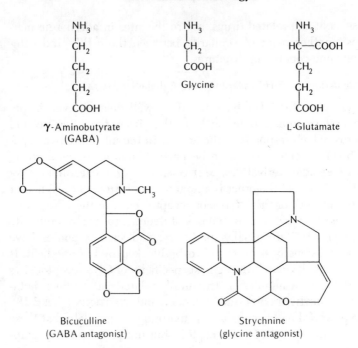

Fig. 2-19   Amino acid transmitter candidates and related drugs.

Drug effects on metabolism

No specific inhibitors of the biosynthesis of any of these amino acids are available. Certain pyridoxal phosphate antagonists, such as THIOSEMICARBAZIDE, inhibit GABA biosynthesis, and this action may be related to the convulsant effects induced by this and related hydrazides, although they are also likely to affect many other metabolic pathways that use pyridoxal phosphate as a cofactor. The metabolic breakdown of GABA by transamination can be inhibited by the compounds D-CYCLOSERINE, AMINO-OXYACETIC ACID, and β-HYDRAZINOPROIONIC ACID, all of which are effective *in vivo* inhibitors, and lead to substantial increases in brain concentrations of GABA. No selective inhibitors of glycine or glutamate metabolism are known, and such compounds would in any case be unlikely to affect only those neurons using these amino acid transmitters since, unlike GABA, glycine and glutamate exist in all cells and are metabolized as part of the free amino acid pool needed for protein synthesis. Specific, high-affinity uptake processes exist in the CNS for all three amino acid transmitters, but so far no selective and potent inhibitors of these uptakes are available.

Drug effects on amino acid receptors

Although the receptors for the amino acids are not well characterized, since they exist only in the CNS, some selective antagonist drugs are available. The convulsant alkaloids, STRYCHNINE and BICUCULLINE (Fig. 2-19), are selective antagonists of glycine and GABA receptors, respectively. Antagonists for the excitatory action of glutamic acid on neurons in the CNS are currently being developed, and various compounds have been reported recently as potential glutamate antagonists.

Other possible transmitter substances

Even if the three amino acids described above are accepted as neurotransmitters, it is likely that there are still other CNS transmitters to be discovered. For example, the nature of the excitatory transmitter released by neurons in any of the primary sensory nervous pathways remains unknown. Thus, we do not know the transmitter in peripheral sensory nerves or in the optic nerve. Among possible candidates for transmitters in these and other CNS pathways are the amino acid ASPARTIC ACID (which has an excitatory action similar to that of glutamate), the nucleotide ATP (for which a transmitter role in the peripheral nervous system in the intestine now seems likely), the amine HISTAMINE (which exists in small amounts in specific locations in the CNS), and small peptides such as SUBSTANCE P (which are known to be present in dorsal roots and other sensory nerves).

CHEMICAL PATHWAYS IN THE BRAIN

Introduction

The concept of chemical transmission in the CNS is a relatively new one. We are only beginning to define the "chemical pathways" in the CNS, in the sense of describing neuroanatomical pathways of neurons with known transmitters. This information, insofar as it is currently available will be summarized for the amine transmitters NE, DA, 5-HT, ACh, and the amino acids GABA and Gly.

In some instances, our understanding of such chemical pathways has progressed rapidly following the development of histochemical techniques for selectively staining neurons that contain particular transmitters. A fluorescence technique pioneered by Hillarp and his colleagues has been used successfully for staining NE-, DA-, and 5-HT-containing pathways. With such methods, the neuron perikarya and fibers with their terminal vesicular stores of specific chemical transmitters can be visualized and their distribution plotted throughout the CNS.

There is still no direct staining technique for ACh, and knowledge of its distribution rests largely on the indirect approach of staining the ACh-hydrolyzing enzyme AChE. In the case of GABA, the evidence for distribution is based mainly on autoradiography. Brain tissue is incubated with radioactively labeled GABA, which is selectively taken up by the GABA-containing neurons. The density of radioactivity in autoradiograms of the tissue identifies these neurons. At present, however, there are no complete maps of the distribution of GABA- or glycine-containing neurons in the CNS.

The distribution of NE, DA, and 5-HT

Fluorescence histochemical technique

Aqueous formaldehyde condensation was first used by Eranko to visualize catecholamines in the adrenal medulla, but Falck

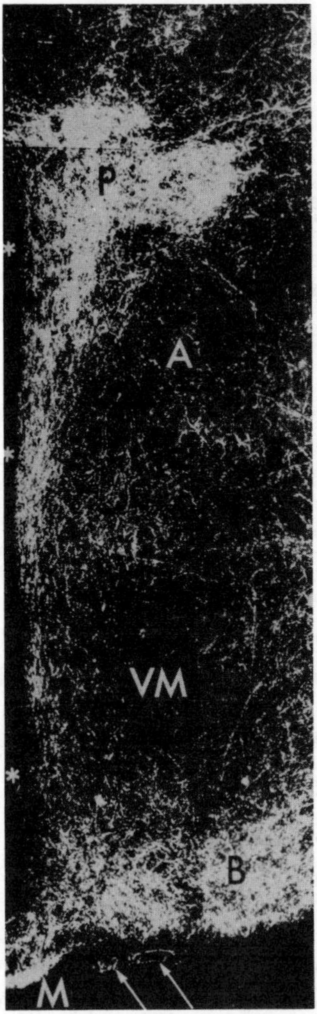

Fig. 2-20 Fluorescent catecholamine-containing nerve terminals in the rat hypothalamus adjacent to the third ventricle, visualized in the fluorescence microscope after exposure of the tissue section to formaldehyde vapor . Magnification, X 200. (From Hokfelt and Ljungdahl, 1972.)

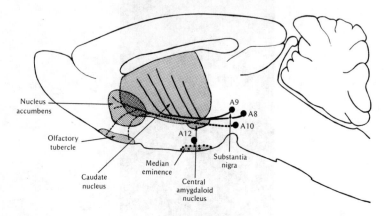

Fig. 2-21 Schematic map of the distribution of dopamine-containing neuronal pathways in rat brain. The cell bodies of these neurons are located in groups A8, A9, A10, and A12, and their terminals are found mainly in the areas of brain indicated by hatching. (From Livett, 1973.)

and Hillarp saw the tremendous potential of the technique and used the highly fluorescent condensation products to plot amine pathways in the brain (Fig. 2-20). The technique depends for its success on rapid freezing of the brain tissue followed by freeze drying at −40° C and subsequent exposure to formaldehyde at 80° C for 1 hour.

The first reaction involves condensation of catecholamines with formaldehyde to give non-fluorescent derivatives (6,7-dihydroxy-1,2,3,4,-tetrahydroisoquinolines). Protein in the tissue then catalyzes the subsequent dehydrogenation of these compounds to yield the corresponding 6,7-dihydroxy-3,4,-dihydroisoquinoline compounds. These products are in a pH-dependent equilibrium with their tautomeric quinone structures, which are responsible for the strong fluorescence. Both NE and DA form compounds that yield green fluorescence on exposure to ultraviolet light, and they are difficult to distinguish by eye. The NE fluoro-

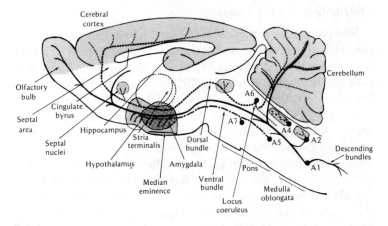

Fig. 2-22 Distribution of norepinephrine-containing pathways in rat brain, as in Fig. 2-21 (From Livett, 1973.)

phore, however, has a labile hydroxyl group in position 4, and, after treatment with hydrochloric acid, its emission peak shifts slightly. This small change can be detected microspectrofluorimetrically. Alternatively, pharmacological treatments, which interfere with one or another of the catecholamines, can be combined with fluorescence histochemistry to visualize NE and DA independently.

Such indolamines as 5-HT also form fluorescent condensation products when exposed to formaldehyde gas, but in this case the yellow fluorescence color is easy to distinguish from the greenish products produced from NE and DA.

Dahlström and Fuxe (1964) were the first to use these techniques to demonstrate the distribution of CNS cell bodies, axons, and terminals that contain NE, DA, and 5-HT. Ungerstedt (1971) more recently has extended such studies and added more details of the terminal distribution of the NE and DA pathways (Figs. 2-21 and 2-22).

Distribution of NE pathways

Norepinephrine terminals in the forebrain originate from neuron cell body groups located in the pons and medulla, which have been designated cell groups A1, A2, A4, A5, A6, and A7. The neurons of the locus coeruleus (A6) have multipolar axons, one branch innervating the Purkinje cells of the cerebellum and others forming a "dorsal bundle" of NE fibers, which terminate in the cortex and hippocampus. The remaining cell groups contribute axons mainly to a "ventral bundle," which inervates the hypothalamus, basal forebrain, and parts of the limbic system. Some of the cell groups, especially A1, also produce descending fibers to the spinal cord, where they terminate mainly in the lateral column in the region of the preganglionic sympathetic neurons. Recently, Olson and Fuxe (1972) re-examined the organization of cell groups A5, A6, and A7 and the fibers arising from them. The dorsal part of A6 is still designated the locus coeruleus, and innervates the hippocampus and cortex, and the ventral part of A6, together with A7, forms the "subcoeruleus" area and gives rise to a fairly thick periventricular plexus along the third ventricle of the hypothalamus and preoptic areas. The NE cell bodies A1 and A2, together with A5, give rise to fibers that innervate the basal and lateral parts of the hypothalamus, preoptic area, and the ventral stria terminalis area. This kind of anatomical detail may seem academic, but when, for example, suggestions are made about the role of the locus coeruleus, it is important to know that, in addition to its innervation of the cortex and hippocampus, this nucleus also innervates the medial hypothalamus.

At the level of the diencephalon, the ascending NE fibers in the dorsal and ventral bundles merge in the medial forebrain bundle, and the fibers then separate to make their discrete terminal innervations.

Additional methods have been employed to verify the observations made with fluorescence histochemistry on tissue from untreated animals. Originally, pharmacological agents that interact with NE were used to decrease or increase the amine content of NE-containing neuronal systems, and the resulting changes in the intensity of fluorescene observed were used to confirm the identity of these neurons. The value of such manipulation is limited because few drugs interact specifically with only one of the amine systems. Of more value has been the method of local injection of 6-hydroxydopamine as pioneered by Ungerstedt (1971). If 6-hydroxydopamine is injected in the vicinity of cate-cholamine-containing neuron cell bodies, their axons, or ter-minals, it is taken up and destroys the neurons. 6-Hydroxydopa-mine can be used to verify the distribution of a particular part of an amine-containing neuronal system if it is injected locally to destroy a discrete part of the system. Standard histochemical fluorescence methods do not give good resolutions of the fine terminals of NE-containing neurons. Recently, two methodologi-cal innovations have improved the visualization of the terminal plexus: (a) an immunofluorescence technique for staining the enzyme dopamine-β-hydroxylase, which is exclusively localized in NE neurons, and (b) the use of glyoxylic acid instead of for-maldehyde as a condensation reagent, which gives rise to fluo-rescent amine derivatives.

The dopamine systems

The DA-containing neuronal systems lie principally in the midbrain anterior to the NE cell bodies. Cell groups A8 and A9 are located in the substantia nigra, and their fibers form the nigro-striatal pathway, which projects together with the NE fibers into the medial forebrain bundle at the diencephalic level. The dopamine fibers leave the medial forebrain bundle more anteriorly to innervate the corpus striatum (caudate nucleus and putamen) and globus pallidus. Cell group A10, which is medial to the substantia nigra, produces an ascending fiber system in-nervating the nucleus accumbens, amygdala, the olfactory tuber-cle and some areas of cortex. Cell group A12 is contained within the arcuate nucleus of the hypothalamus, and the short axons of these neurons innervate the median eminence. Also, DA-containing neurons are found in the amacrine cell layer of the retina.

The contribution of the fluorescence histochemical method to our knowledge of neuroanatomy is well illustrated by the discovery of the nigro-striatal DA pathway. Although this neuronal system contains about three-quarters of all the DA in the brain, the fibers are extremely small, and their existence had not been detected with classical silver-staining histological methods. After the histochemical demonstration of this pathway with fluorescence, more refined modifications of the Nauta silver-staining techniques were used to demonstrate fibers from the substantia nigra to the striatum. Experiments also indicate that this major chemical pathway has an important role to play in motor integration (Ungerstedt, 1971); it is doubtful whether it would have been discovered without this sophisticated chemical mapping approach.

Distribution of 5-HT

The location of 5-HT neurons and their fiber and terminal systems in the rat brain were described initially by Dahlström and Fuxe (1964). In succeeding years, the 5-HT system received less attention by anatomists, than the NE and DA systems.

In the rat, the 5-HT-containing neurons are located in the nuclei of the raphe system situated dorsally near the midline of the brain stem. They extend from the raphe pallidus nucleus in the caudal medulla to the raphe dorsalis nucleus in the caudal mesencephalon. Some 5-HT cell groups are located more laterally in the paragiganto cellularis nucleus and in the ventral part of the area postrema. At least some of the ascending 5-HT fibers to the forebrain travel in the medial forebrain bundle. The terminals of the 5-HT axons innervate the pontomesencephalic reticular formation, hypothalamus, lateral geniculate nuclei, amygdala, pallidum system, hippocampus, anterior hypothalamus, and preoptic area and cortex. The raphe 5-HT neurons also send descending fibers to the spinal cord.

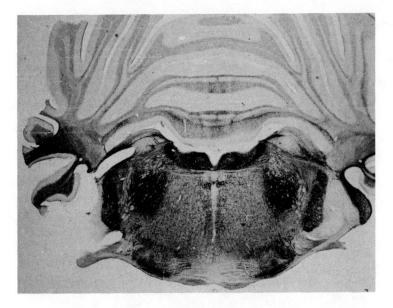

Fig. 2-23   Section of rat brain stem stained for acetylcholinesterase. Note intense staining of oculomotor nuclei in the brain stem and the relatively weak staining of the overlying cerebellum. (Kindly supplied from unpublished results by Dr. P. Lewis, Physiological Laboratory, University of Cambridge.)

The 5-HT neuronal system of the cat brain has been studied in detail and is essentially similar to that of the rat. It is in the cat that functional evidence was obtained of a crucial role for the raphe 5-HT system in sleep processes (Jouvet, 1972).

Distribution of cholinergic neurons

Shute and Lewis (1967) made use of the AChE-staining technique for the detailed mapping of cholinergic pathways in the cat CNS (Figs. 2-23 and 2-24). Their original maps remain the

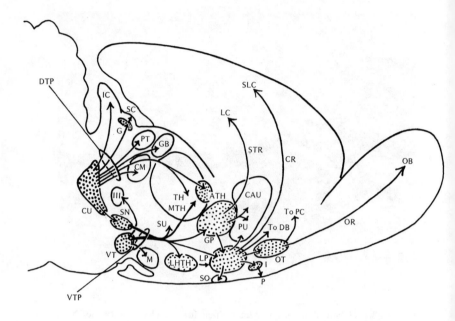

Fig. 2-24 Cholinesterase-staining neurons (probably cholinergic) in rat forebrain. Neuron cell bodies in various nuclei (stippled areas) send axons (arrows) to terminate in various forebrain regions. Abbreviations: ATH, antero-ventral and antero-dorsal thalamic nuclei; CAU, caudate; CM, centromedian (parafascicular) nucleus; CR, cingulate radiation; CU, nucleus cuneiformis; DB, diagonal band; DTP, dorsal tegmental pathway; G, stratum griseum intermediale of superior colliculus; GB, medial and lateral geniculate bodies; GP, globus pallidus and entopeduncular nucleus; I, islets of Calleja; IC, inferior colliculus; III, oculomotor nucleus; LC, lateral cortex, LHTH, lateral hypothalamic area; LP, Lateral preoptic area; M, mammillary body; MTH, mammillothalamic tract; OB, olfactory bulb; OR, olfactory radiation; OT, olfactory tubercle; P, plexiform layer or olfactory tubercle; PC, precallosal cells; PT, pretectal nuclei; PU, putamen; SC, superior colliculus; SLC, supero-lateral cortex; SN, substantia nigra pars compacta; SO, supraoptic nucleus, STR, striatal radiation; SU, subthalamus; TH, thalamus; TP, nucleus reticularis tegmenti pontis (of Bechterew); VT, ventral tegmental area and nucleus of basal optic root; VTP, ventral tegmental pathway. (From Shute and Lewis, 1967.)

most comprehensive description of the ACh systems, if one accepts the enzyme stain as a reliable indicator of cholinergic neurons. In this technique, the brain is perfused *in vivo* with formaldehyde and then sectioned on a freezing microtome. Alternate sections are incubated with butyrylthiocholine as a substrate for non-specific pseudocholinesterase or acetylthiocholine together with a specific pseudocholinesterase inhibitor to demonstrate true AChE. The sections are then treated with copper sulfate and sodium sulfide, which stain enzyme-active sites black. Since AChE is distributed throughout the neuron, it is impossible to determine from any given section whether stained axons are efferent or afferent to a given brain structure. Lewis and Shute, however, discovered that AChE activity changed in different ways on the two sides of a cut axon. The enzyme accumulated on the cell body side of a cut and disappeared on the terminal side. The combination of selective lesions with the enzyme-staining technique helped in plotting the neuronal pathways. So did biochemical assays for choline acetyltransferase, the enzyme concerned in the synthesis of ACh, which is an exclusive marker for cholinergic neurons. After lesions to a cholinergic pathway, the activity of both AChE and choline acetyltransferase fell in a parallel manner. With this combination of techniques, for example, the cholinergic input to the hippocampus via the fornix was demonstrated.

There are two main cholinesterase-containing pathways projecting to the rat forebrain. The dorsal tegmental pathway arises mainly from the nucleus cuneiformis situated in the dorsolateral part of the mesencephalic reticular formation and ascends to innervate the tectum, pretectal area, geniculate bodies, and thalamus. The fibers of the ventral tegmental pathway arise from the substantia nigra and ventral tegmental area of the midbrain and innervate the basal forebrain areas from which additional AChE-containing neurons project to all regions of the cerebral cortex and olfactory bulb. These pathways are considered part of the ascending reticular formation and are implicated in arousal. Unfortunately, AChE is not exclusively limited to the synaptic region of cholinergic neurons. It is present in the cell bodies, the axons and synaptic terminals of cholinergic neurons, and it may also be present in the cell membranes of neurons that receive a cholinergic input, especially in the bodies and dendrites of such cells. Thus, AChE-staining of cell bodies can yield a misleading picture and cannot be used as the sole criterion that a neuron is cholinergic. For example, the noradrenergic cell bodies of the locus coeruleus stain intensely for AChE, as do the noradrenergic neurons of peripheral sympathetic ganglia, yet they are almost certainly not cholinergic neurons.

It is likely that reliable histochemical or immunochemical methods for localizing choline acetyltransferase will be developed in the future, and these should provide less ambiguous maps of cholinergic pathways, since there is little doubt that this biosynthetic enzyme is strictly localized to cholinergic neurons.

Distribution of GABA and glycine

These two amino acids seem to be the most important inhibitory transmitter substrates in the mammalian CNS. Little is known, however, of the pathways in which they are used. Glycine acts only in the spinal cord and lower brain stem as an inhibitory transmitter. It seems to be localized in the spinal cord in small inhibitory interneurons located in the medial gray matter and projecting to motor neurons and other cells in the ventral horn. There is, however, no histochemical procedure that allows such neurons to be visualized directly. Glycine neurons possess a specific high affinity uptake process for glycine, and this may permit the development of autoradiographic techniques to visualize such neurons after they have been labeled with radioactive glycine.

The identity and distribution of GABA neurons is similarly unknown at present. Biochemical estimations and neuropharmacological evidence suggest that in the spinal cord GABA is largely confined to nerve terminals in the dorsal horn. In supraspinal regions, GABA is present in substantial concentrations in nearly all gray matter, where it is probably the major inhibitory substance. Few long-axon pathways involving this transmitter have been described, however. Although histochemical procedures for visualizing sites of GABA metabolism have been developed, these are not considered reliable indicators for GABA-containing neurons. Autoradiographic techniques are being developed, based on the existence of specific high affinity uptake sites for labeled GABA in neurons using this transmitter. Such autoradiographic studies at the electron microscope level have indicated that, in many regions of the brain, GABA may be the transmitter in up to one-third of all the synaptic terminals. Biochemical findings after various experimental lesions suggest that some long-axon pathways containing GABA may exist. There is good evidence that the Purkinje cells of the cerebellum and their axons, terminating in the various cerebellar nuclei, use GABA as their transmitter. Lesion studies also indicate the existence of a pathway of GABA-containing fibers from the globus pallidus and other striatal regions terminating in the substantia nigra, which contains the highest density of GABA terminals in the brain.

Until reliable autoradiographic methods or immunochemical techniques, perhaps based on localizing the GABA biosynthetic enzymes glutamic decarboxylase, are available, little progress can be made in detailed mapping of the GABA pathways.

③ | Determinants of Drug Action

Dose-response relations and mode of administration

It is not adequate in behavioral pharmacology to study the effect of a single dose of a drug on a complex behavior. As the dose of drug is increased, a point is reached where any behavior is depressed. At doses below this point, the drug may stimulate or disorganize the ongoing behavior, but, in many cases, the effective dose range producing this effect is narrow and easily missed unless a wide range of doses is studied. This is a hard lesson to learn because, when one considers many of the classical pharmacological systems for quantifying drug action, such as isolated smooth muscle (cf. Fig. 2-1), the response varies in a graded manner with increasing dosage. In such preparations, the dose-response curves tend to be simple, and, since there is only a single variable (e.g., contractility) to be influenced by the drug, interpretation of the results is easy. Other physiological responses, however, are, like behavior, determined by several interacting variables. For example, if the activity of drugs that change blood pressure is to be understood, their effects on all the interacting variables must be considered. Of course, it is only a matter of technical competence to investigate the effects of various doses of a drug on a variety of behavioral parameters; the more difficult task is to select the parameters to be studied.

In studying psychoactive drugs, there is a tendency to think that all behavioral effects are mediated by effects of the drug on the brain. Systemically injected drugs may, however, have pronounced peripheral as well as central effects, and the possibility that behavioral effects are secondary to changes in peripheral physiology should be considered. For example, isoprenaline is an agonist at β-adrenoceptors. Intravenous injections of small doses of isoproterenol (4 μg) induce drinking behavior. The drug releases renin from the kidney, which promotes the formation of angiotensin in the blood, and this peptide passes the blood-brain barrier and induces drinking by stimulating a site in the preoptic region of the hypothalamus. In the rat, the injection of 40 μg of isoproterenol into the preoptic region induces drinking, and this result has been used to support the hypothesis that there are β-adrenoceptors in the brain involved in the induction of drinking. It is probable, however, that after such a large intracerebral injection a sufficient amount of isoproterenol could leak from the brain to the systematic circulation to induce renin release and that drinking was a result of this peripherally mediated effect rather than of any direct action of isoproterenol on the brain. This is supported by the observation that surgical removal of the kidney abolishes isoproterenol-induced drinking irrespective of the route of drug injection. Peripheral drug effects may also serve as discriminative stimuli for behavior. Cook et al. (1960) describe experiments in which dogs were set up in restraining harnesses and their respiration, heart (EKG) and intestinal activity, and leg withdrawal recorded. l-Epinephrine (10 μg/kg), l-norepinephrine (10 μg/kg), or ACh (20 μg/kg) were infused intravenously, and, 30 seconds after the injection, the leg was shocked and the withdrawal reflex observed. Leg withdrawal within 30 seconds of the injection prevented the shock. No other stimuli preceded the shock, and, yet, after a certain number of training trials, successful avoidance occurred with all the injected substances.

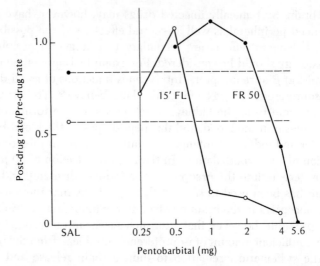

Fig. 3-1 Effect of pentobarbital on pecking behavior of pigeons. Log dose-response curves. Each point represents the arithmetic mean of the ratios for the same four birds at each dosage level on each schedule. Open circles, mean effects, birds working on 15 FI; solid circles, birds working on FR 50; dotted lines, control response levels; SAL, after saline injection. (Reproduced from Dews, 1955a.)

ONGOING BEHAVIOR AS A DETERMINANT OF DRUG ACTION

Schedule of reinforcement

Reinforcing events are the major determinants of ongoing behavior, and a given drug can produce very different effects depending on the precise nature of such reinforced behavior. Drugs that increase behavior show these effects most clearly. Dews (1955a) was the first to recognize the schedule of reinforcement as the most important determinant of drug action. He reported that the behavioral effects of the barbiturate, pentobarbital (1

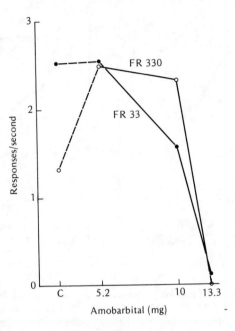

Fig. 3-2 Dose-response curves for amobarbital at two parameter values of fixed-ratio reinforcement (FR). Each drug point is the average number of responses in a 10-minute session starting 15 minutes after drug injection. Notice that after 10 mg of amobarbital, the curve for FR 33 is depressed below its control value, and the curve for FR 330 is elevated above its control value and also above the FR 33 curve. (Reproduced from Morse, 1962.)

mg), in pigeons depended on the operating schedule of reinforcement. For example, fixed-interval responding was markedly reduced by this dose of the drug, whereas FR 50 responding was increased (Fig. 3-1). At this dose of pentobarbital, there is no obvious physical disability, and, yet, "by use of these techniques a behavioral effect of a drug can be detected." Similarly, Morse (1962) showed that another barbiturate, amobarbital, at a dose of 10 mg/

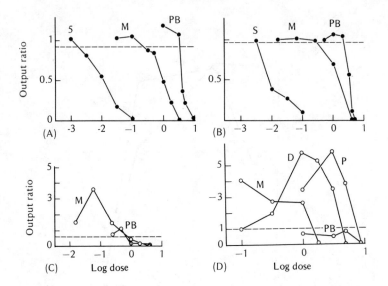

Fig. 3-3 Effect of drugs on performance on various schedules. (A) 1 VI;
(B) FR 50; (C) 15 FI; (D) FR 900. (Output ratios are calculated for
whole experiments, not just the first 15 minutes.) S, scopolamine; M,
methamphetamine; PB, pentobarbital; D, *d*-amphetamine; P, pipradol.
The filled-in circles above and the open circles below are to emphasize the
change in scale of the ordinate between the upper pair and the lower pair.
(Reproduced from Dews, 1958.)

kg increased FR 330, while decreasing FR 33 in the pigeon (Fig.
3-2).

In a subsequent study, Dews (1958) compared pentobarbital
with three stimulant drugs, methamphetamine, *d*-amphetamine,
and pipradol. Again pentobarbital further increased the already
high rates of FR responding in addition to VI and FI responding, while depressing FR 900 performance. The amphetamines,
however, gave the opposite pattern of results, markedly increasing FR 900 and FI 15 responding and barely increasing the
FR 50 or VI 1 base lines (Fig. 3-3).

Determinants of Drug Action

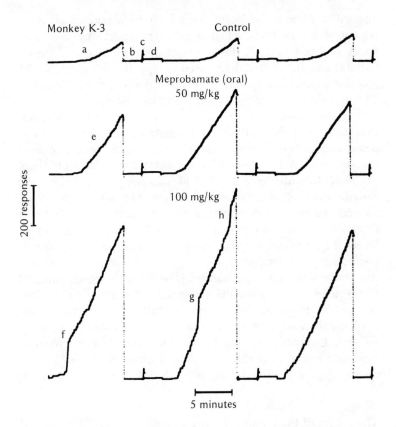

Fig. 3-4 Effects of meprobamate on a squirrel monkey's behavior maintained by a multiple schedule of food reinforcement, including FI-10 (a), FR-30 (c), and TO-2.5 (b and d) components. The recording pen reset to the bottom of the record when reinforcement occurred. (From Cook and Kelleher, 1962.)

Multiple schedules provide a powerful technique for demonstrating schedule control of drug effects. Instead of studying FI and FR performance independently, a multiple schedule can be used in which a fixed-ratio requirement alternates with a fixed-interval condition. Distinctive visual stimuli signal which component of the multiple schedule is operating at any one time. Using such a base line, the effects of amphetamine and pentobarbital can be clearly dissociated. Amphetamine increases FI and decreases FR responding, whereas pentobarbital depresses FI responding and leaves FR performance intact.

It is also possible to use more complex multiple schedules. Cook and Kelleher (1962), for example, described a four-component schedule under the discriminative control of four visual stimuli. A 10-minute FI was followed by 2.5 minute time-out with no reinforcement; a FR 30 followed that, and the cycle ended with another 2.5 minute time-out (Fig. 3-4). Such schedules can be used to demonstrate the considerable specificity of drug action. The minor tranquilizer, meprobamate, at a dose of 50 mg/kg increased terminal rates of responding during the FI component without increasing FR rates or inducing responses during the time-out. Discrimination between the conditions and of the temporal relationship within the FI was normal. At 100 mg/kg of meprobamate, however, although discrimination between the four elements remained, discrimination within the FI was disrupted, and bursts of high responding occurred at random times during the interval and often in the initial segments when response rates are normally very low.

The nature of the reinforcer

It is commonly assumed that the nature of the reinforcer maintaining behavior is the most important determinant of any effect drugs may have on that behavior. Contrary to this belief, there is a growing realization that, first, relationships between stimuli and their reinforcing potential are not rigid, and, second, the important thing is not the nature of the event that follows behavior but rather the way the event is programmed in relation to behavior.

Food and water reinforcement are most commonly used in behavioral pharmacology, but intracranial self-stimulation (which in some way mimics the cues associated with natural reinforcement) and heat (Weiss and Laties, 1961) can also be used to maintain identical patterns of responding. A drug like chlorpromazine will produce a very similar dose-dependent depression of behavior maintained by any of these reinforcers.

It is not difficult to accept the common behavioral property of positive reinforcers, but it is important to realize that negative reinforcers also share this common behavioral property. For example, shock is called an aversive stimulus, but when programmed on an avoidance or escape schedule, it increases rates of responding.

It is striking that the reinforcers food and escape from shock can be programmed to produce indistinguishable patterns of responding (Fig. 1-6). To illustrate this point, Kelleher and Morse (1964) present cumulative records of lever pressing in squirrel monkeys maintained either on a multiple FI/FR for food or for shock-escape. It is well known that amphetamine increases FI and reduces FR responding for food, and, despite the opposite direction of the behavioral changes, the anorexic effect of the drug has been used to explain the depression of FR responding. The observation that FI/FR responding for food or shock-escape is changed in an identical manner by amphetamine undermines any motivational interpretation of the action of the drug (Fig. 3-5).

Chlorpromazine also affects behavior maintained under the two conditions of motivation in an identical manner. There may be drugs that affect behavior maintained by positive and negative reinforcement in different ways, but, as far as studies of the major classes of psychoactive drugs are concerned, the schedule of reinforcement rather than its nature is the more important determinant of drug action. If the generated pattern of responding is identical, so is the drug response. In the past, however, quantitative differences in drug response have been reported for

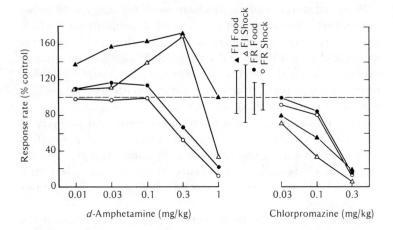

Fig. 3-5 Effects of *d*-amphetamine sulfate and chlorpromazine hydrochloride on rates of responding under multiple FI FR food and shock schedules. Three monkeys were studied on each multiple schedule. Each drug was given intramuscularly immediately before the beginning of a 2.5-hour session. At least duplicate observations were made in each monkey at each dose level; thus, each point is based on six observations or more. Summary dose-response curves for the four-component schedules were obtained by computing the means of the percentage changes in average response rates from control to drug sessions. The dashed line at 100% indicates the mean control level for each component. The vertical lines in the middle of the figure indicate the ranges of control observations expressed as a percentage of the mean control value. Note the general similarity of the pairs of dose-effect curves for fixed-interval and fixed-ratio components. (Reproduced from Kelleher and Morse, 1964.)

positively and negatively maintained behavior. Wenzel (1959) trained cats in the presence of a stimulus to press a lever for food and in the presence of a different stimulus to press another lever to avoid electric shock. Reserpine increased response latencies (i.e., time to move the lever) more for responses to the stimulus associated with shock than to the stimulus associated with food, but, as Dews and Morse (1961) comment, control response latencies were longer to start with in the shock condition. Cook and Kelleher (1962) report that chlorpromazine decreased food-reinforced responses at doses lower than those required to affect responses that postponed electric shock. They used a concurrent schedule on which each response postponed a shock by 30 seconds and every 100th response was reinforced with food. Just after a food reward, the response rate was controlled by the shock contingency and was 0.1 response/second. As the next food reward approached, this contingency controlled behavior and the response rate increased to 1.0/second. In this study, the positive and negative reinforcement did not control identical response patterns, and, thus, different drug responses would be expected. (The general importance of an ongoing rate of responding as a determinant of drug response is discussed later in the chapter.) In contrast, when the same shock is programmed as an immediate consequence of behavior it acts as a punisher and decreases responding. Such observations make it clear that the unpleasant nature of the stimulus is secondary, and, more importantly, they undermine the use of such hypothetical intervening variables as "fear" or "anxiety" to explain the effects of shock. The same shock should create the same fear, and yet the elicited behavior can be in opposite directions. The concept of fear and fear motivation requires considerable expansion to explain such effects of shock stimuli.

Discriminative stimuli as determinants of drug action

A discriminative stimulus is one in the presence of which an animal is reinforced (S^D) or not reinforced (S^Δ). Such stimuli can be used to modulate responding in very specific ways, and certain drugs have been shown to selectively modify this control. Many classes of drug have an effect on discriminative control, but, in most cases, this effect is only one of a wide spectrum of behavioral effects and, therefore, does not characterize the drug.

As we shall see, however, the phenothiazines are an exception to this rule. Their effect on discriminative control has proved valuable both in differentiating phenothiazines from other drugs such as reserpine, that also have a generally depressant effect on behavior, and in differentiating among the various phenothiazines (Cook and Kelleher, 1962).

Discriminative stimuli may be exteroceptive (e.g., visual or auditory stimuli) or interoceptive (e.g., autonomic responses, time cues). Interoceptive cues have not received much attention. This is unfortunate because there is every reason to suppose that these cues are extremely important in determining drug responses; they are after all the autonomic and, therefore, invariant stimulus corollaries of drug action. Particularly important is the possibility that interoceptive cues associated with drug injections may be as important in determining the behavioral response to the drug on that *and subsequent* occasions (Overton, 1966) as any specific effects it may have on the CNS. By comparison, the external stimulus environment is somewhat arbitrary. The blood pressure response to epinephrine is invariant, although the environmental conditions under which the drug is taken may vary each time.

Fig. 3-6 (A) Diagram showing sequence of stimuli in the various schedules used. R, B, Y, and W indicate that the red, blue, yellow, and white lights, respectively, were on behind the key. (B) Effect of pentobarbital on performance on schedule 1. Ordinate and abscissa scales have been superimposed on an original record. The short diagonal lines on the original record show when the rewards occurred. Below the record is a key showing the nature of the stimuli throughout the run. The conventions in the key are the same as those of Fig. 6-1. Note the almost complete absence of responding in the S— periods and the lack of effect of 3 mg pentobarbital (PB) on performance on this schedule. (C) Effect of pentobarbital on performance on schedule 4. Note the almost complete absence of responding in the S— periods before the drug, but the large number of responses in the second S— period after the drug. Performance in the S+ periods is not obviously affected by this dose of pentobarbital. (Reproduced from Dews, 1955b.)

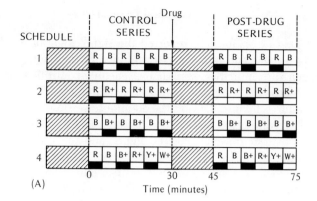

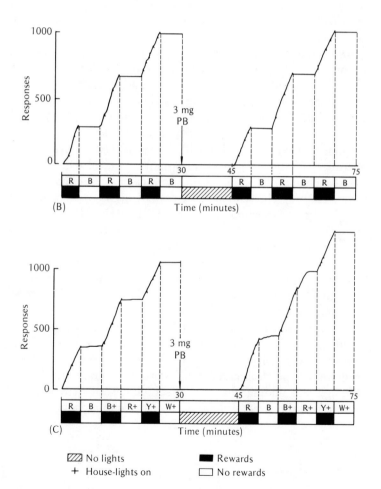

| ▨ No lights | ■ Rewards |
| + House-lights on | □ No rewards |

Dews (1955b) first reported the significance of exteroceptive visual cues and how drugs could modify the control exerted by such discriminative stimuli on schedule-controlled responding. Pigeons were trained to peck an illuminated key on a VI 1-minute schedule. During the 30-minute session, S^D (S^+) and S^Δ (S^-) periods alternated. The response key was illuminated with one of four different colored lights, and the house light in the testing chamber was either on or off. These stimuli could be combined to form eight discrete discrimination stimuli, and six of them were used as the S^D and S^Δ stimuli. Four schedules were studied; on three of them single S^D and S^Δ alternated; on the fourth the stimuli were conditional, e.g., the house light was either combined or not combined with red for S^D and S^Δ stimuli, and, in addition, none of the stimuli were repeated within the session (Fig. 3-6). Phenobarbital was one of the drugs studied, and it was found that a dose of 3 mg/kg had no effect on S^Δ responding on schedules 1-3 but markedly increased S^Δ responding on schedule 4. Dews concluded that the more complex the discriminative control the more likely it is to be disrupted.

Chlorpromazine is a drug that alters discriminative control regardless of the complexity of stimulus control. On a simple FI/FR schedule, chlorpromazine results in a flattening of behavior control. The scalloped FI pattern becomes a steady low rate throughout the interval, and the characteristic high FR rates are reduced. These changes are often considered to reflect a loss of discriminative control, but, on this basic schedule, such a loss cannot be differentiated from the general depressant effects of chlorpromazine on all response patterns. The same criticism can be applied to the study of Blough (1957), in which pigeons were trained on a conditional discrimination to peck the darker of two keys when a vertical bar between the keys was illuminated, and the lighter key when it was not. Two measures of performance were observed: the total response output and the accuracy of the discrimination. Chlorpromazine lowered both, although the finding that the effect on discrimination lasted longer than the general depression of responding suggests that the two effects may be dissociable. Vaillant (1964) achieved such a dissociation by using a more complex discrimination schedule with pigeons. Two keys were simultaneously illuminated, one with blue and the other with red light. The schedule was arranged so that at the start of the session only pecks on the blue key were reinforced on a FR 30 schedule for six consecutive reinforcements. Then, without any exteroceptive cue, reinforcement became available on the red key, where pecks were reinforced on a FI 300 schedule four times. The FR/FI sequence was repeated three times, and thirty reinforcements were given. Chlorpromazine (10 mg/kg) did not change the *total* output of responses during the FI sequences (i.e., pecks to red key plus erroneous pecks to blue key). If the pecks to the separate keys were analyzed, however, it was found that the drug increased pecking to the blue FR key during the FI sequences, while simultaneously reducing pecking to the red FI key, which was actually being reinforced at that time.

The specificity of stimulus control can be demonstrated with stimulus generalization methods (see Fig. 1-8). Use of this method is limited to stimuli that belong to identified physical continua. When an animal is under the control of more complex stimuli, such as visual patterns, or, more importantly, the whole constellation of environmental cues encountered under normal conditions, the experimenter is at a loss to know how to vary the stimuli systematically. Stimulus generalization and discrimination methods provide a potentially powerful way of finding out exactly how a stimulus appears to an animal under the influence of a drug, although as yet these methods have not been fully exploited in behavioral pharmacology. In the studies reported to date, several drugs have been shown to modify generalization gradients, but in no case has this proved to be a unique effect of the drug class in question. Hearst (1964), who pioneered these studies, reports that D-amphetamine, scopolamine, and caffeine all modify generalization gradients to a range of lights varying in brightness.

Terrace (1963) discovered another important feature of stimulus control when he observed that the method of acquiring a discrimination influenced its susceptibility to drug action. Pigeons learned a horizontal/vertical discrimination where they were exposed to the S^D and S^Δ throughout training or when the S^Δ was introduced initially as a weak physical stimulus and only gradually achieved equal intensity with the S^D. In the former condition, errors were made to the S^Δ during learning; in the latter, the tendency to respond to the S^Δ was very weak, and learning, therefore, occurred without error. Imipramine and chlorpromazine had no disruptive effect on discrimination achieved by errorless learning but had a marked effect if errors had been made during acquisition. Under the drug, the birds made a high number of erroneous responses to the negative pattern.

As far as interoceptive cues are concerned, the most attention has been given to the role of temporal cues as discriminative stimuli. Sidman (1956) was one of the first to recognize the value of differential reinforcement of low rates of responding (DRL) schedules for studying timing cues. In the DRL procedure, an animal must space his responses in time. For example, on 20-second DRL, a lever press produces a reinforcement only if 20 seconds or more have elapsed since the preceding response. If a response occurs too soon, the DRL timer is reset, and the timing interval begins anew. The frequency distribution of time intervals between successive responses (interresponse times) illustrates the accuracy of timing that develops on DRL schedules.

Amphetamine increases the frequency of short inter-response times, and this disrupts DRL performance; with appropriate methods of analysis, it can be shown that any disruption of temporal control is secondary to the more basic response-stimulating effect of amphetamine. By contrast, it can be shown that the effects of chlorpromazine on schedules involving temporal discrimination are much more closely tied to sensory control (Weiss and Laties, 1964a). Pigeons were trained on an FI 5-minute

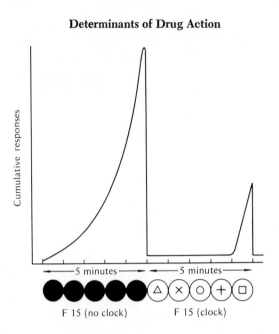

Fig. 3-7 Symbols used during the clock and no-clock conditions. During the no-clock condition the key was illuminated by a red light. The cumulative records above the symbols represent typical performance during the two conditions. (Reproduced from Weiss and Laties, 1964a.)

schedule. Then, on alternate intervals, an external visual "clock" was superimposed, and discrete form stimuli appeared on the response key during successive segments of the FI (Fig. 3-7). The pigeons watched the "clock" when it was present and achieved even better controlled scalloped response patterns on the FI. Under amphetamine only the "no clock" FI performance was disrupted; in the presence of the clock, the disruptive influence of the drug was attenuated (Fig. 3-8A). Chlorpromazine, however, disrupted the pattern of responding under both conditions, suggesting that neither intero- nor exteroceptive cue could control behavior in the presence of this drug (Fig. 3-8B). Specific evidence of an effect of chlorpromazine on the discrimination of

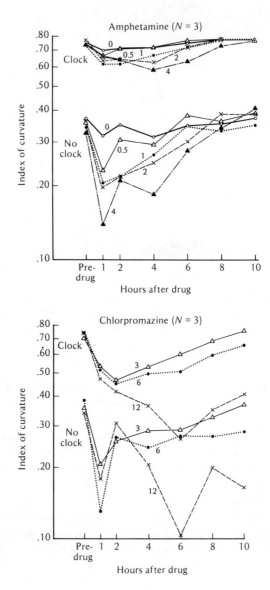

interoceptive cues comes from a study of Cook et al. (1960), in which dogs no longer showed conditioned leg avoidance to injections of NE after a dose of 50 μg/kg of this phenothiazine.

Punishing procedures as a determinant of drug action

If an unpleasant stimulus, such as a shock, is unavoidable, the effect on behavior is quite different from that seen if the same shock is used as a negative reinforcer. Punishing stimuli that are programmed to occur following responses suppress behavior severely, and *immediate punishment* procedures of this kind have been very useful in characterizing drug effects. The Geller procedure, a concurrent VI for food, with every response simultaneously punished, can be used to illustrate the fact that, although certain psychoactive drugs are insensitive to the nature of the reinforcer, they are influenced by whether reinforcement or punishment is operating. Amphetamine, for example, which invariably increases reinforced responding, further decreases punished responding regardless of how the punishing stimulus is scheduled. Another example is provided by such minor tranquilizers as chlordiazepoxide, which strongly increases the rate of punished responding although it has weak rate-increasing effects on behavior maintained by reinforcers (Geller and Seifter, 1960; Geller et al., 1962).

On the Geller-Seifter procedure, the responses of the animal initiate the punishment stimuli. If these stimuli are programmed to occur irrespective of the animal's behavior, suppression is less complete. There is some evidence that the tranquilizing drugs,

---

Fig. 3-8 (A) Index of curvature during the clock and no-clock conditions after different amounts of amphetamine sulfate. (B) Index of curvature during the clock and no-clock conditions after different amounts of chlorpromazine hydrochloride. The numbers adjacent to each curve indicate the dose in milligrams per kilogram. (Reproduced from Weiss and Laties, 1964a.)

which release shock-suppressed behavior, act less potently if such adventitious punishment has been used. Basic behavioral studies of immediate and adventitious punishment procedures have existed for a number of years, and it would be most interesting to see some quantitative assessment of, for example, the effect of tranquilizing drugs on behavioral base lines maintained with these two punishment procedures.

One of the punishment procedures most extensively used in behavioral pharmacology is the Estes-Skinner procedure. Different studies have produced a confusing array of results with this procedure, and these results would not, on their own, have revealed how crucial punishment is in determining drug action. Reserpine, morphine, and meprobamate have been claimed by some to restore responding during the preshock stimulus and by others not to. The results with this procedure illustrate the necessity of defining the operating behavioral variables in any procedure before using it to characterize drugs. Further study of the Estes-Skinner procedure itself has shown that, under certain conditions, responding may increase during the preshock stimulus, and, even when suppression occurs, its degree depends on: (a) the duration of the pre-shock stimulus, suppression being greatest with short stimuli; (b) the schedule of reinforcement used to maintain responding; (c) the experimental history of the animal.

Since these variables are themselves determinants of drug action, irrespective of their interaction with response-suppression, it is not surprising to find that the Estes-Skinner procedure has yielded conflicting results.

Rates and pattern of ongoing behavior as determinants of drug action

Dews drew attention to the importance of rate of responding as a determinant of the action of certain classes of drugs. In the study referred to earlier, in which four different schedules of reinforcement were studied (Dews, 1958), amphetamine increased responding where the base-line activity was low and had no effect on or decreased high base lines. This was interpreted in terms of drug effects on inter-response times.

Analysis of the changing response rate during FI performance provides another way of getting at this problem. FI reinforcement generates an escalating response rate over the time interval: a low rate immediately after the reinforcement and a high rate as the next reinforcement approaches. This cumulative record of FI performance is therefore "scalloped"; under amphetamine, the scallop becomes a linear increase. Several workers have measured response rates in the consecutive segments of the FI, and an analysis of the effect of amphetamine shows a clear relationship to the different base-line rates during the various segments. Kelleher and Morse (1968) have analyzed the effect of amphetamine in this way on FI/FR shock avoidance behavior in the squirrel monkey. Amphetamine illustrates the rate dependency most clearly. Barbiturates also show the effect on low base lines (Fig. 3-9) but reduce high rates of responding less dramatically than amphetamine (Dews, 1964). The minor tranquilizers, meprobamate and chlordiazepoxide, are more like amphetamine but have not been intensively studied.

This important principle is not widely referred to, and, yet, a cursory inspection reveals that it is obeyed with amphetamine-induced stimulation when ICS, food, water, temperature presentation, postponement of electric shock, termination of loud noise, and termination of shock are used to maintain *low* rates of ongoing behavior. Similarly, irrespective of the reinforcer, high rates of responding are insensitive to amphetamine.

Multiple schedules that juxtapose low and high rates of responding demonstrate this very clearly. Using FI/FR multiple schedules of food or shock-escape reinforcement in the squirrel monkey, Kelleher and Morse (1964) show that 0.3 mg/kg D-amphetamine almost doubled response rate on FI while almost halving FR responding (Fig. 3-5). In the rat, Clark and Steele

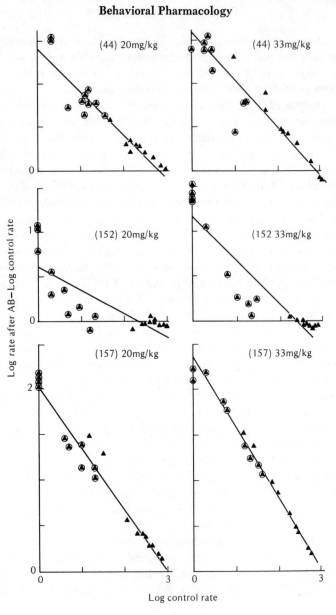

(1966) used a three-component schedule: a 4-minute period with no reinforcement followed by a 4-minute FI, in turn followed by three reinforcements under an FR 25 schedule. After amphetamine they consistently found increased responding in the first two segments and decreased responding in the third segment.

Punishment, as we have seen, also generates low rates of responding, but it seems that the releasing effect that such drugs as the minor tranquilizers have on punishment are not entirely explicable in terms of rate-dependency. If matched rates of responding are generated by a multiple FI food, FI punishment schedule, chlordiazepoxide and meprobamate increase responding more in the VI punishment segment than in the food-reinforcement segments, indicating a unique relationship between tranquilizers and punishment, which is independent of their rate-increasing effects (McMillan, 1973a).

General environmental conditions as a determinant of drug action

In operant conditioning situations, the aim is to study the effect on behavior of a few variables that are under experimental con-

---

Fig. 3-9   Dependence of the effect of amobarbital (AB) on the pre-drug rate of key pecking in the pigeon. *Abscissa:* log of rate as responses per session (total of 500 seconds, since each 25-second period occurred once in each of twenty cycles); *ordinate:* change in log rate following amobarbital, intramuscularly. Since the 500-second interval was divided for recording purposes into twenty periods of 25 seconds, there are twenty points on each graph, ten representing periods when the light was on (circled triangles) and ten representing periods when the light was off (triangles). The line through the points was calculated by least squares from all points. On the ordinate are plotted all points where the mean rate of responding was 1 or less response/500 seconds; this arbitrary assignment makes possible the logarithmic plot. Exclusion of these indeterminate points would not appreciably affect the regression line. (Reproduced from Dews, 1964.)

trol and to eliminate all other variables. The success with which this is achieved determines the significance of the results, and the same is obviously true of behavioral pharmacology. It is impossible to identify and control all the specific and non-specific environmental conditions that could influence the drug/behavior interaction. But the importance of controlling such factors as far as possible is illustrated by the results of experiments in which unspecified environmental influences have been shown to influence drug effects dramatically.

Amphetamine toxicity is one example. Amphetamine in sufficiently high doses will kill rodents, and the pharmacological measure of these lethal doses is the LD_{50} (the dose killing 50% of the animals within a specified time interval). Amphetamine has a significantly lower LD_{50} in rodents housed in overcrowded conditions than in their normally housed litter mates (15 mg/kg instead of 111 mg/kg). A similar result can be obtained by exposing rodents to shock, stress, noise, or raised temperature.

A second example is afforded by Steinberg and her associates (Rushton and Steinberg, 1964) who report that the spontaneous motor behavior seen in a Y-maze is increased by amphetamine if the rats are inexperienced in the situation but that the effect is lost if the rats are experienced.

Although it is possible, for experimental purposes, to isolate and study intero- or exteroceptive discriminative cues, the total environment determining drug action under natural conditions presents a far more complex picture. The experiments of Schachter and Singer (1962) illustrate this very well. Students were asked to take an injection of a harmless substance in a study of its effect on vision. The drug was epinephrine, and some subjects were correctly told that it would produce transient side effects, including hand tremor, increased heart rate, and facial flushing. Others were given inaccurate details of the likely side effects, including foot numbness, itching, and headache. While they were waiting for the drug to take effect, the subjects in both groups were with an individual who had been instructed to indulge in such foolish behavior as playing basketball with scrap paper and flying paper airplanes. The behavior of the drugged subjects was noted, and it was found that the correctly informed group was relatively unaffected by the stooge's behavior, whereas the misinformed subjects exhibited active emotional involvement, joined in raucous behavior with the stooge, far outdoing the excesses of the mysterious stranger. The same physiological background produced by the drug, combined with identical behavior on the part of the stooge, resulted in quite different behavior in the two groups, apparently entirely as a function of what they had been told about the effects of epinephrine.

IMPORTANCE OF THE VARIOUS DETERMINANTS FOR DISTINGUISHING DRUG CLASSES

There are clearly many determinants of drug action, and all of them should be studied in order to characterize any particular drug fully. The hope is that in this way different classes of psychoactive compounds may be distinguished and the ways in which they influence behavior defined. This has not been achieved, but some examples will be given of how certain drug groups may be characterized by applying the methods of behavioral analysis we have described.

Analgesics

Morphine and barbiturates are prescribed for the relief of intractable pain. Weiss and Laties (1958) have used an ingenious titration method for determining shock threshold to measure the increase in pain threshold after morphine injections (see Chapter 4). Studies of shock-punished behavior, however, make it clear that a change in pain threshold is not sufficient to alleviate pain in all situations, and, indeed, that reinstatement of behavior

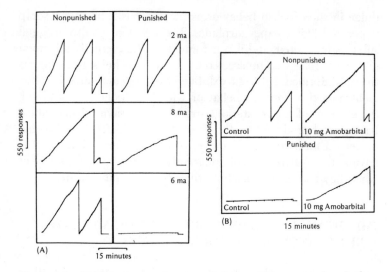

Fig. 3-10 (A) Representative cumulative response records of three pigeons for daily sessions on Mult VI VI+ punishment. The nonpunishment and punishment components of the schedule alternated every 4 minutes. *Left:* nonpunishment periods; *right:* punishment periods. The diagonal marks on the records show food deliveries. Each response during the punishment periods produces a 25-msec electric shock of the current indicated. Suppression during the punishment components varies among the birds. (B) Cumulative response records of one pigeon for a control and drug session on Mult VI VI+ punishment. *Left:* control records; *right:* drug records for the following day. The shock current during the punished components was 6 ma, which greatly suppressed the level of responding. After 10 mg amobarbital, the level of nonpunished responding is somewhat decreased (top right), whereas the level of punished responding is greatly increased (bottom right). (Reproduced from Morse, 1964.)

suppressed by shock is not likely to be mediated by such a mechanism. Although morphine markedly increases pain thresholds, it will not, for example, reinstate behavior suppressed by punishment. In a typical experiment, pigeons were trained in the presence of an orange light for five reinforcements under an FR 30. The light was then changed to white, and, although

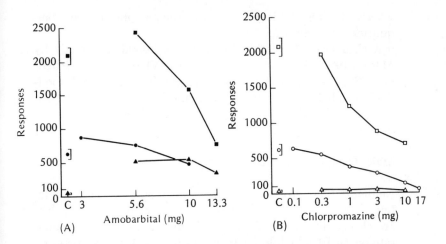

Fig. 3-11 (A) The dose-effect curve for amobarbital on punished responding for three pigeons. (B) The dose-effect curve for chlorpromazine on punished responding for three pigeons. (Reproduced from Morse, 1964.)

the FR 30 was still in operation, every tenth response was punished (Kelleher and Morse, 1964). Behavior in the white light was suppressed, and morphine did not reinstate it.

In contrast, barbiturates resulted in an immediate reinstatement of the punished responding, and further evidence that this was not related to an analgesic effect was afforded by the observation that if shock was omitted suddenly in undrugged sessions, behavior was reinstated but less quickly than after barbiturates. Morphine and barbiturates clearly act to relieve the anxiety associated with pain in different ways.

Major vs. minor tranquilizers

Minor tranquilizers (barbiturates in small doses, meprobamate, and benzodiazepines) potently release punished responding, whereas the phenothiazines and other neuroleptics (major tranquilizers) are totally ineffective.

A clear example of this dissociation is found in a study by Morse (1964). Using a multiple VI food/VI punishment schedule (Fig. 3-10), he found that amobarbital increased food-reinforced behavior marginally and punished behavior markedly, whereas chlorpromazine produced a dose-dependent decrease in both behaviors (Fig. 3-11).

Major tranquilizers vs. stimulants

Neither of these groups of drugs attenuate punished responding, but, if they are tested on reinforced patterns of behavior, they are clearly differentiated. Amphetamine increases the response rate on an FI schedule for food and for shock-escape, whereas chlorpromazine decreases both behaviors (Fig. 3-5) (Kelleher and Morse, 1964).

Minor tranquilizers vs. stimulants

Barbiturates in small doses and benzodiazepines have a rate-increasing effect on food-reinforced behavior. The effect is strong in the case of the barbiturates, and, here, they are difficult to distinguish from stimulants. If punished responding is studied, however, they are clearly dissociable; amphetamine is ineffective in restoring punished responding, whereas the barbiturates are highly effective. This example illustrates how drug groups may share a certain property that is primary to one and secondary to the other and how this is only appreciated if they are compared on several behavioral parameters.

Antidepressants vs. other drug groups

Antidepressants are easily distinguished from stimulants by their failure (except in pigeons and dogs) to increase rates of reinforced behavior. They are also clearly distinguishable from minor tranquilizers because they do not attenuate punished responding. Unfortunately, however, they are extremely difficult to dissociate behaviorally from the major tranquilizers. This is a disconcerting failure of behavioral pharmacology, considering the markedly different therapeutic uses of these drug groups.

The major tranquilizers, like the antidepressants, have rate-increasing effects in pigeons and dogs and do not attenuate punished responding. Only by indirect methods that probably depend on the different neuropharmacological actions of the drugs can these groups be dissociated. Amphetamine-induced locomotor activity, for example, is potentiated by antidepressants of both the tricyclic and MAO inhibitor classes, and this behavior is blocked by major tranquilizers. Similarly, antidepressants, but not chlorpromazine, potentiate the increased rates of responding for intracranial self-stimulation induced by amphetamine.

Indirect methods are perfectly valid in behavioral pharmacology, but it is important to try to develop direct tests to characterize the two major classes of psychoactive drugs that do not reliably increase any behaviors yet studied. Baltzer and Weiskrantz (1970) report an ingenious step in this direction with a potential test for antidepressants involving the Crespi effect (Chapter 1, p. 53).

If an animal that is responding for a regular-sized reinforcement suddenly receives a much larger or smaller one, the rate of ongoing behavior increases or decreases; it is suggested that this reflects "elation" or "depression." It will be interesting to observe the effect of antidepressants on this sensitive base line, which may reflect yet another important effect of reinforcement contingencies.

4 | Drugs and Behavior

A very wide range of substances have pronounced effects on behavior. Not surprisingly, the drugs that have been used clinically to manipulate the physiological state of the brain in normal subjects, e.g., anesthetics and pain killers, or to alleviate behavioral disorders, e.g., tranquilizers and antidepressants, and those taken by otherwise normal people to induce pleasant psychological changes, e.g., alcohol, nicotine, hallucinogens, etc., have been

TABLE 4-1
BEHAVIOR AND DRUGS TO BE STUDIED

1. Arousal	Stimulants, e.g., amphetamines Sedatives, e.g., barbiturates, alcohol
2. Learning and memory	Protein synthesis inhibitors Steroids

3. Mood	Antidepressants:
	    Tricyclic, e.g., Imipramine
	    MAO inhibitors, e.g., Iproniazid
	    Opiates, e.g., morphine

4. Anxiety	Minor tranquilizers:
	    Benzodiazepines, e.g., chlordiazepoxide
	    Meprobamate

5. Psychosis	Neuroleptics, e.g., chlorpromazine, haloperidol Hallucinogens, e.g., LSD, *Cannabis*

the most systematically studied. Furthermore, the drugs used in psychiatry have received the most attention. We propose to restrict our discussion to the major groups of drugs that influence five selected aspects of behavior, as shown in Table 4-1.

In each section a description of the basic neuropharmacological properties of the drug group precedes a discussion of its effects on behavior.

AMPHETAMINES AND RELATED COMPOUNDS

Classification

Amphetamine (Fig. 4-1) has several effects upon behavior. In particular, it is a stimulant, and it is also an anorexic, i.e., it suppresses appetite for food. The d-isomer of amphetamine (DEXE-DRINE) is more potent in both respects than the l-isomer and is the form of the drug commonly used. Such related compounds as D-METHAMPHETAMINE ("SPEED") (Fig. 4-1A) are even more potent stimulants of behavior, and "rigid" analogues, in which the side chain is cyclized, such as METHYLPHENIDATE and PIPRADOL, appear to stimulate behavior in a manner very similar to that of amphetamine. Other derivatives, however, are very weak stimulants, while retaining the anorexic effects of amphetamine, e.g., CHLORPHENTERMINE, PHENMETRAZINE (PRELUDIN), and FENFLURA-MINE (Fig. 4-1B). The latter drugs are used clinically as appetite suppressants and have less of the undesirable stimulant and sleep-disrupting properties of amphetamine itself.

Neuropharmacological properties

The amphetamines are an important group of drugs to neuro-pharmacologists because their mode of action is fairly clearly de-

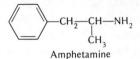

Amphetamine

STIMULANTS

ANOREXICS

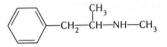

Methamphetamine

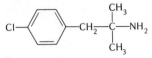

Chlorphentermine

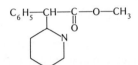

Methylphenidate

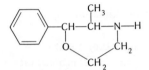

Phenmetrazine

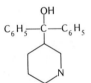

Pipradrol

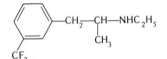

Fenfluramine

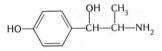

p-Hydroxynorephedrine
(amphetamine metabolite)

Fig. 4-1 Amphetamine and related compounds.

fined. Amphetamine is an indirectly acting sympathomimetic amine in peripheral adrenergic systems, that is, it mimics the effects of norepinephrine (NE) by displacing this amine from peripheral adrenergic nerve endings, although amphetamine itself has little or no direct effect on adrenergic receptors. The drug appears to act similarly in the brain, where it has been shown to release both NE and dopamine (DA) from nerves containing these amines. The fact that the powerful central stimulant activity of amphetamine is not shared by other indirectly acting sympathomimetic amines may be explained simply by the ease in which amphetamine penetrates into the brain compared with other amines of this type that are less soluble in lipids (cf. Chapter 2). The notion that amphetamine acts by displacing catecholamines from storage sites in the brain is strongly supported by the finding that pretreatment with drugs that inhibit catecholamine biosynthesis, α-methyl-p-tyrosine, for example, completely prevents amphetamine stimulation of behavior. On the other hand, amphetamine continues to stimulate animals in which brain catecholamines have been greatly depleted by reserpine treatment. This can be explained, however, if it is assumed that amphetamine releases the catecholamines from the small pools of newly synthesized amines that are still present after reserpine treatment. In addition to causing catecholamine release, amphetamine is also a potent inhibitor of the NE- and DA-uptake systems in adrenergic terminals, and this inhibition tends to enhance and prolong the effects of the amines released by the drug by blocking their normal inactivation by these systems.

The behavioral stimulant actions of amphetamine are abolished in animals treated with 6-hydroxydopamine; this effect is only seen, however, if massive depletions of both DA and NE have been achieved. In rats treated with intracerebral injections of 6-hydroxydopamine shortly after birth, a very extensive destruction of both NE and DA can be achieved; such animals, when adults, do not respond to amphetamine. Less substantial catecholamine depletions caused by 6-hydroxydopamine in adult animals are rarely sufficient to impair amphetamine responses.

The release of brain catecholamines by amphetamine is usually not sufficient to reduce the normal brain concentrations of these amines, although depletion of NE does result after treatment with large doses of amphetamine. This is because resynthesis of catecholamine normally proceeds so rapidly that the amine displaced by amphetamine is rapidly replaced. A rapid depletion of both catecholamines is seen, however, if amphetamine is given in conjunction with an inhibitor of catecholamine synthesis, such as α-methyl-p-tyrosine. Further evidence that the action of amphetamine depends upon the activation of central adrenergic mechanisms comes from the finding that the behavioral action of the drug is specifically antagonized by such drugs as chlorpromazine, which block catecholamine actions at noradrenergic and dopaminergic receptor sites in the CNS.

Stimulation of behavior by amphetamine and related substances

Arousal is probably the most important general variable determining the behavioral responses of animals. Most animals have a diurnal pattern of sleeping and waking, but, during the waking phase, when animals respond to the external environment, a wide range of arousal levels may exist. A variety of physiological and psychological variables determines the mean level of arousal at any one time, probably by interacting with the reticular activating system of the brain. Malmo (1959) has suggested that there is a U-shaped relationship between the physiological state of arousal and behavioral efficiency. If the arousal level is too low, there is virtually no behavior, and, when the optimum level is exceeded, arousal results in a general disruption of behavior.

Many drugs affect arousal as part of their psychopharmacological profile; the mood-changing opiates, for example, may also stimulate or depress other facets of behavior, whereas the antipsychotic, chlorpromazine, has the additional property of depressing all forms of behavior. There are drugs that principally affect arousal, which are used clinically or socially for this reason. The amphetamines will be considered in this context.

One of the most marked behavioral effects of amphetamine is its ability to stimulate various categories of spontaneous motor behavior in all the species that have been studied. A variety of automatic recording devices have been used for quantifying locomotor activity, including running wheels, jiggle cages, photocell devices, circular runways, and electromagnetic movement registering systems (Animex). When interest focused on the effect of arousal-inducing stimuli in the environment on locomotor activity, a variety of situations were devised for varying the nature of such stimulation. These include Y-maze situations with feeding troughs in the arms (Kumar, 1969), boxes with interesting objects placed in them (Carlsson, 1972), operant situations in which a lever press initiates a change in an environmental stimulus, such as a light or, as in the case of Butler's famous monkey experiment, the opening of a window on an interesting vista.

Amphetamine has been shown to increase behavior in all these situations. For a number of years, such results have been interpreted simply as evidence of the stimulatory action of the drug. Direct somatomotor facilitation may indeed underlie the running activity seen when a rat is given amphetamine in a familiar environment. Normally an animal is inactive in such an environment, and the drug induces a short-lived burst of running. It has been appreciated recently that, in many of the more complex environments used for assessing motor behavior, the recorded activity reflects the interaction of responses to several different aspects of the environment. For example, a rat moves about a wire cage resembling its home cage in a certain way, but it behaves in quite a different way if interesting objects are placed on the floor of the cage. Ambulation is usually the measure taken, presumably because it is easy to record. But not enough attention has been given to the consideration that, in different situations, this mean level of activity reflects the response to several interacting aspects of the environment. Amphetamine increases activity in all situations, but it is important to specify which aspect of locomotor behavior (e.g., activity related or unrelated to an investigation of interesting objects) has been changed by the drug.

Berlyne (1955) was one of the first to recognize this point, and he devised an ingenious apparatus to identify motor responses to different aspects of the environment. Robbins and Iversen (1973) have used this apparatus to quantify locomotor behavior in the large area of a box against responses to interesting objects placed in an alcove at one end of the box. Normal animals distribute their behavior between these two features of the environment in a correlated fashion. After amphetamine, a marked increase in locomotor activity in the large area is seen in conjunction with reduced attention to the localized stimuli. Similar observations have encouraged the belief that amphetamine reduces exploration of the environment; it is more likely, however, that the effect of the drug is not directly to reduce exploration but that reduction of exploration occurs as a consequence of a direct stimulation of locomotion in the main cage. The suggestion is that amphetamine increases the probability of certain responses to the disadvantage of others and that where the opportunity for running exists its probability of occurrence is greatly increased by low doses of amphetamine. In addition to identifying and quantifying component behaviors in any situation, it is important to recognize that these elements of the motor repertoire may well not be equally sensitive to pharmacological agents. For example, running wheels are often used for quantifying locomotion, but activity in this situation reflects drug stimulation in an unpredictable and different manner to that observed when animals are in simple wire cages. First, among rats there are "wheel runners" and "non-runners," and, despite their low basal activity, the latter do not respond to amphetamine. Second, although runners do respond, their activity in the wheels tends to increase over several consecutive test days, even in the absence of the drug. The rats apparently learn to run. It has been suggested that activity levels in wheels depend on proprioceptive feedback. Whether or not this is so, base-line running wheel activity is a labile base line for drug studies and could not be expected to show the same drug sensitivity as other measures.

The maximum locomotor response in photocell cages is elicited by a dose of d-amphetamine of 1.5 mg/kg in the rat. If the dose is increased to 5 or 10 mg/kg, lomocotor stimulation is no longer seen, and stereotyped behavior emerges. Stereotypy refers to a behavioral state when isolated elements of the normal behavioral repertoire, which seem quite inappropriate in the particular environment, are constantly repeated. The number of elements of behavior that occur during stereotypy is reduced as the dose of the drug increases. In the rat, for example, stereotyped locomotion, sniffing, neck movements, and rearing are seen in weak stereotypy responses, but when these become intense, gnawing occurs to the exclusion of virtually all other behavior. Schiørring (1971) has also stressed that increasing doses of amphetamine produce a progressively more intense stimulation of fewer and fewer categories of behavior. At low doses, locomotion and full body movement are stimulated; at 5 mg/kg, locomotion is not seen, but sniffing, licking, and biting are observed. In the most intense stereotypy, biting and gnawing predominate.

Conditioned response patterns are affected in much the same way as unconditioned behavior by amphetamine. The characteristic pattern of responding under fixed-interval schedules of reinforcement is stimulated by amphetamine (Dews, 1955b). The low rate of responding immediately after a reinforcement is particularly sensitive to the rate-increasing effect of the drug. In contrast, the high rates at the end of the interval show less increase and indeed may even be depressed, as are the high rates of responding seen on fixed-ratio schedules.

On the basis of such results, Dews (1958) has proposed a "baseline" theory of the stimulant action of the drug: that low rates of ongoing behavior are stimulated relatively more than high. An analysis of the increase in responding relative to base line in the sequential segments of the fixed interval supports this proposition.

In reviewing the effects of amphetamine on behavior more than 10 years ago, Dews and Morse (1961) suggested that: "All these findings are compatible with the view that an important determinant of the effects of the amphetamine is the control rate of responding per se, irrespective of species, or type of motivation, or response studied." Whereas the rate of ongoing behavior is a major determinant of amphetamine action, it is clearly not the only factor. In several different experiments, amphetamine has failed to increase low rates of ongoing behavior and, in other situations, the stimulatory action of the drug is associated with disruption rather than facilitation of performance. Lyon and Randrup (1972) have proposed that response topography should also be considered in relation to the stimulatory action of amphetamine. One of their experiments illustrates the point elegantly. Groups of rats were trained on one of two shock reinforcement schedules. One group was required to make a discrete lever press to turn off a shock and to further delay (and thus avoid) subsequent shocks. The other group was required to hold the lever depressed to escape and avoid shock. The effect of 1 to 5 mg/kg of d-amphetamine was studied on these two behavior patterns. A dose of 1 mg/kg increased lever pressing and lever release as part of the general stimulatory action. As a consequence, avoidance was facilitated on the lever-press schedule and was disrupted on the lever-hold schedule. In contrast, the stereotyped behavior induced by 3 and 5 mg/kg d-amphetamine tended to "immobilize" animals in the vicinity of the lever and disrupted lever-holding behavior less than lever-pressing responses. The authors propose that amphetamine may disrupt or enhance responding depending on the compatibility of the response with elements of behavior stimulated by amphetamine. Dews (1958) had earlier proposed that behavior occurring at a low rate is more likely to be increased by amphetamine than that at a high rate. Lyon and Randrup view this base-line effect as secondary to response compatibility, since the very low rates of responding on the lever-hold schedule was not increased by stimulatory doses of amphetamine if the stimulated responses were incompatible with the conditioned response.

It is surprising how many of the apparently anomalous effects of amphetamine can be explained by consideration of the baseline effect and response compatibility. For example, amphetamine has been reported to facilitate acquisition and performance in certain learning tasks, particularly shock-avoidance. Kulkarni and Job (1967) refer to earlier studies and also report acquisition of a bar-pressing avoidance response in a Skinner box to be greatly enhanced by 1 mg/kg d-amphetamine. A 15-second light/sound stimulus signaled the approaching shock, which could be avoided by a lever press. The higher mean avoidance level achieved under the drug could still be demonstrated 1 week after treatment. There was no evidence that the effect was related to suppression of freezing behavior in the shock situation, as previously suggested by Kriekhaus et al. (1965). An explanation in terms of a general increase in "somatic motor activity" was also discounted, since the time course of the two effects differed, and no increase in activity was observed in the inter-trial intervals when the light/sound stimulus was absent. Rech (1965) has emphasized that the basic tendency of rats to be "good" or "bad" avoidance performers also determines the potency of amphetamine in facilitating performance. Consistently poor performers showed the greatest improvement, but the effect clearly had not been on acquisition because, when the drug was discontinued, their performance regressed to its originally poor level. It seems unlikely, however, that there is any unique relationship between amphetamine and avoidance behavior. In both of these experiments, the avoidance response was not well developed before the drug treatment, and it is likely that improvement occurred because the response stimulation produced by the drug was compatible with the required avoidance response. When avoidance-responding is firmly established and trained to a high criterion, no improvement is seen with amphetamine, and the drug has instead been reported to disrupt both active and passive shock-avoidance. One is forced, therefore, to seek alternative explanations for these avoidance learning results, and, in this context, the suggestion of Lyon and Randrup (1972) is most important.

Whereas the stimulatory effect of amphetamine on unconditioned and simple reinforced behavior and the apparently discordant facilitory and disruptive effects on certain other behaviors are well encompassed by the base-line theory, tempered by considerations of response compatability, there are categories of behavior that respond to amphetamine in ways that cannot be so obviously accommodated. The effect of amphetamine on behavior suppressed by punishment is one such example. Immediate punishment, if superimposed on a bar-pressing response for food, severely depresses that response. Although the rate of responding is low in the presence of punishment, amphetamine will not reinstate behavior suppressed in this way. Indeed, if anything, amphetamine augments the suppression. This result has been obtained in several species and has encouraged one recent experimenter to comment: "it is clear that some other factor modifies the usual rate-dependent effects of d-amphetamine when responses are punished" (McMillan, 1973a).

The clear dissociation of the effects of amphetamine on reinforced and punished responding may lend further support to the notion that these procedures represent opposite ways of controlling behavior. Before accepting this explanation, however, the effect of amphetamine on punished responding requires further examination in relation to the base-line theory and response compatibility. It could be argued that the effect is compatible with the classical stimulatory effect of amphetamine, which increases the emission of the most probable response in any situation. Training determines that probability. With traditional schedules of reinforcement, responding is probable, whereas after punishment not responding is the appropriate behavior. In both situations, amphetamine intensified these tendencies, in one to increase and in the other to decrease absolute response rates.

It has also been claimed that amphetamine changes the discriminative control of sensory stimuli over behavior. The reports on discrimination behavior are apparently as contradictory as those on avoidance behavior. Dews (1955b) studied the effect of methamphetamine on responding controlled by discriminative stimuli of varying complexity (Fig. 3-3). Under the influence of the drug, the simpler single stimulus S^D/S^Δ control was maintained, whereas discriminative control by the more complex stimuli (schedule 4) was disrupted, and a marked increase in responding to the S^Δ occurred. At the same time, Sidman (1956) reported that amphetamine disrupted performance on a schedule where low rates of responding are required (DRL), and temporal discrimination is thought to be involved. More responses occurred, and their inter-response time was short, a response strategy that prevents reinforcement. Glick and Jarvik (1969) found, in monkeys, that the accuracy of visual matching to sample of colors was decreased by amphetamine. It seems likely that these effects on discriminative control may be secondary to the response-stimulating effect of amphetamine, whereby the emission of irrelevant responses interferes with discriminatively controlled response patterns. It is also possible that, in these situations, the strength of the discriminative control ultimately determines the degrees of disruption. Where such control is relatively weak, the behavior is liable to be disrupted by non-specific response increases. This explanation could be entertained in all the examples cited. With complex discriminative cues, S^Δ responding is not as precisely controlled as when simple cues are operating (Dews, 1955b). But DRL performance requires discrimination, which is notoriously difficult for animals to achieve, for a strong response tendency has to be overcome (Sidman, 1956); in the matching to sample task of Glick and Jarvik (1969), the accuracy of matching behavior was poor even in the absence of the drug.

In contrast, amphetamine is reported to improve discrimination under certain conditions. Gendreau et al. (1972) have studied in man the effect of 0.25 mg/kg methamphetamine on acquisition of the eyelid response to a puff of air, under classical conditioning procedures to 1500 Hz (CS+) and 500 Hz (CS—) tones. Under the drug, the accuracy of the discrimination improved largely because fewer responses were made to the unreinforced stimulus (500 Hz, S—). It has been suggested by Hill (1970) that certain stimulants, such as amphetamine and pipradol, facilitate behavior because they intensify the control of behavior by discriminative stimuli of both the intero- and exteroceptive kind. Reinforcing stimuli, whether unconditioned like those associated with food and water or conditioned like the noise associated with the presentation of food in a Skinner box, gain in facilitory control over behavior. In support of this position, Hill (1970) reports an experiment in which rats were treated with pipradol or saline, and then bar-pressing behavior was extinguished in the presence or absence of a conditioned reinforcer. Pipradol greatly enhanced extinction response rates in the presence of the CR and decreased rates in the absence of the stimulus. Clearly, more experimentation is required to determine whether these effects on discriminative control are another facet of the facilitatory property of amphetamine or represent an independent effect of the drug.

Another unconditioned behavior influenced by amphetamine is eating. Indeed, the potent anorexic effect of the drug constitutes its principal therapeutic use. This is generally recognized to be an effect of the drug independent of the modulating influence on conditioned behavior described above. Yet the doses of amphetamine that reduce food intake also stimulate conditioned responding for food and lack of appetite clearly cannot explain why animals respond avidly for food reward. Certain areas in the hypothalamus are known to be a focus for the control of food-intake behavior. Direct application of the neurotransmitter NE to the preoptic region of the hypothalamus induces eating and satiety. It is generally thought that the NE-releasing properties of amphetamine underlie the anorexic effect, although there is considerable disagreement about the precise nature of the mechanism (discussed in Iversen and Iversen, 1974).

Amphetamines provide the best example of how the neuropharmacological effects of a drug may be related to a range of behavior mediated (in all probability) at different sites in the nervous system and involving different neurochemical substrates. The dopaminergic system of the striatum plays a central role in amphetamine-induced stereotypy, whereas both NE and DA appear to be involved in locomotor stimulation. The role of these two amines in the stimulation of conditioned behavior remains to be explored. Although a release of hypothalamic NE is thought to underlie the appetite-suppressant effects of amphetamine, Ungerstedt's observation (1971) of anorexia after selective lesions of the nigro-striatal dopaminergic pathway suggests that dopaminergic systems may also be involved in some critical manner in the broad control of feeding behavior.

BARBITURATES

Classification and neuropharmacological properties

There are many different barbituric acid derivatives with sedative properties. They range from drugs with slow metabolism and long duration of action, such as PHENOBARBITAL, to drugs with ultra-short actions, such as THIOPENTAL. Before the advent of the minor tranquilizers, drugs like phenobarbital were widely used as anti-anxiety agents and were given in small doses to reduce emotional tension and produce mild skeletal muscle relaxation. The barbiturates, however, readily lead to addiction and tolerance when used chronically. The risk of accidental poisoning or suicide is also much greater than with the newer anti-anxiety drugs, and thus barbiturates have fallen out of favor for psychopharmacological use.

Within the brain, barbiturates produce a number of effects, in particular a general slowing of oxidative metabolism and a depression of synaptic transmission. These effects do not appear to be confined to any particular neuronal system. There is thus no evidence for a selective action of any of these drugs, and it is possible that their action is related to an over-all depressant effect on brain metabolism and activity.

Behavioral pharmacology

In large doses barbiturates suppress ongoing behavior and induce sleep. But in small doses they increase rather than decrease behavioral output, and this facilitatory effect may well be related to their value as anxiety-reducing drugs.

Dews (1955a) reported that pentobarbital increased response rates in pigeons working on a multiple FI/FR schedule of reinforcement. The FI performance was more sensitive than FR responding to the rate-increasing effect of barbiturates. The facilitation seen with small doses may be associated with improved discriminative behavior in certain circumstances. This may be a result of the drug's ability to modulate sensory input, by acting on the reticular activating system, and, thus, maintaining a level of arousal optimal for behavioral efficiency. An interesting example of this effect of barbiturates is their reported ability to improve impaired *delayed response* performance in monkeys with lesions of the frontal lobe (Wade, 1947). It has been suggested that these lesions disrupt the normal inhibitory control exerted by the frontal cortex over the hindbrain reticular activating system. The resultant disinhibition of sensory arousal mechanisms produces a highly distractable animal that is unable to perform well on certain delay tasks. Barbiturates are thought to overcome this difficulty by attenuating sensory input. Weiskrantz et al. (1965) have reported that the minor tranquilizer meprobamate improves delayed response behavior in monkeys with frontal lobe lesions to the same degree as pentobarbital.

It is notable that, even with depressant doses of barbiturates, responses to simple discriminative stimuli in the environment remain unimpaired, despite general motor depression and ataxia.

Pigeons on an FI/FR schedule, with red and blue lights used as the stimuli associated with the two schedules, will, under a large dose of barbiturate, appear grossly incoordinated and ataxic in the Skinner box. Nevertheless, when the colored light indicating that FR performance is demanded comes onto the key, they will struggle to the key and respond quickly with the required number of pecks.

This is the case only when relatively simple levels of stimulus control are operating. Dews showed, for example, that when red and blue S^D and S^Δ alternated during a fixed-interval schedule, pentobarbital (3 mg/kg) left discrimination performance intact. If, however, there was a different S^D and S^Δ stimulus during each segment of the FI, and discrimination accordingly became more difficult, the same dose of pentobarbital disrupted discriminative control, and considerable responding during the S^Δ was seen (Fig. 3-6).

This is further supported by the observation that monkeys on a difficult size discrimination task and pigeons on a conditional brightness discrimination task (Blough, 1957) show decreased accuracy of discrimination after pentobarbital. This cannot be attributed to a depressant effect of the drug because, in the latter experiment, increased response rates were associated with the impaired accuracy of discrimination. The temporal discrimination required for successful performance on DRL schedules is also severely disrupted by pentobarbital. Not all CNS depressants have this effect; ethanol, for example, although it generally depresses responding, leaves temporal discrimination unaffected (Sidman, 1956).

Delay discrimination tasks reveal another feature of depressants—although the registration of information may be impaired by the drug, its subsequent retrieval may be enhanced. During the delay, irrelevant stimuli are normally responded to, and interference occurs. The longer the delay, the greater the interference and, consequently, the poorer the retention. Depressants in small doses depress the arousal mechanism, which not only impairs registration but also reduces the level of interference.

Jarvik (1964) found this to be the case in monkeys trained on a 1- or 8-second delayed response task. The accuracy was reduced by pentobarbital, but the normal deterioration in performance as the delay lengthened was eradicated. Summerfield (1964) described impaired registration and improved retention in man using the gaseous anesthetic nitrous oxide as the depressant.

The apparently paradoxical ability of depressants and stimulants at some doses to facilitate and at others to impair behavior is conveniently illustrated by an inverted U-shaped relationship between behavioral efficiency and arousal. A particular level of arousal is optimal for any particular behavior. Barbiturates in small doses increase specific arousal by eliminating irrelevant stimuli but eventually depress arousal. Amphetamine progressively increases arousal, until eventually the level is so high as to be incompatible with efficient behavior. It is, therefore, possible for either depressants or stimulants to enhance behavioral efficiency by inducing the optimum level of arousal. But when a particular element of behavior is performed efficiently, the prediction is that further increases in the dose of either class of compound will eventually disrupt behavior; depressants because of anesthesia and stimulants because of over-arousal.

The similarity of the facilitation seen with both amphetamine and the barbiturates is further emphasized by the finding that the rate-increasing effects of both drugs are related to the level of ongoing behavior. Indeed, Dews (1964) was the first to formulate the base-line phenomenon on the basis of studies of the effect of amobarbital on FI behavior in the pigeon. If successive segments of the fixed interval are examined, barbiturates and amphetamine increase low rates of responding in the initial segments and decrease high rates of responding in the terminal segments.

The stimulatory property of these drugs explains their use for inducing "high" states in man, and both barbiturates and amphetamines are drugs of abuse. Tolerance is observed with both types of drug, and this has been verified in animal experiments. It is suggested that the arousal-inducing function of both groups of drugs is mediated at the level of the reticular-activating system. There is electrophysiological support for this in the case of the barbiturates, and the fact that amphetamine excites many neurons in the reticular-activating system, when iontophenetically applied, encouraged Bradley (1968) to make the same claim for amphetamine.

Potentiation between amphetamines and barbiturates

When these drugs are given in combination they potentiate the rate-increasing effects. Rushton and Steinberg (1964) reported that naive rats in a Y-maze showed greater stimulation after a combination of amphetamine (0.75 mg/kg) and amobarbital (15 mg/kg) than after either drug alone. Since rats experienced in the situation did not show such effects, the authors suggested that these drugs result in stimulation by reducing fear, which would presumably be at a much higher level in naive rats. An alternative explanation could be that the low level of spontaneous behavior in naive rats, unlike the higher levels in experienced animals, is increased by amphetamine and low doses of barbiturates. Rutledge and Kelleher (1965) favor such an interpretation, having shown similar potentiation of the rate-increasing effects by amphetamine and barbiturates in pigeons pecking on a multiple FI/FR schedule of reinforcement. In neither of these schedule conditions, could fear be proposed as an intervening variable, and yet the drugs given singly or in combination increased low rates of responding in the early part of the FI and did not affect the high levels of responding characteristic of the FR schedule.

The contrasting effects of barbiturates and amphetamines on punished responding

The similarity of the effects of amphetamine and barbiturates on unconditioned and reinforced behavior may be contrasted with their dissimilar effects on punished responding. Whereas amphetamine generally intensifies the effect of punishment, bar-

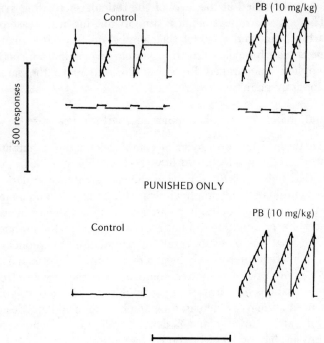

Fig. 4-2 Effects of pentobarbital (PB) on key pecking suppressed by punishment. Each frame shows a complete control session followed by a complete drug session. The drug was given intramuscularly 15 minutes before the beginning of the drug sessions. *Upper:* in nonpunishment components (event record displaced upward), a 30-response, fixed-ratio schedule of food presentation was in effect in the presence of an orange light. The termination of each nonpunishment component is indicated by a small arrow. In punishment components (event record displaced downward), a 30-response, fixed-ratio schedule was in effect in the presence of a white light; each of the first ten responses of each ratio produced a 35-msec electric shock of 6 ma, 60 cycles ac, delivered through gold wire electrodes implanted around the pubis bones of the bird. The termination of each punishment component is indicated by the resetting of the pen to the bottom of the record. *Lower:* the punishment procedure was in effect throughout each session in the presence of a white light. Note that under both procedures pentobarbital attenuates the suppression of responding by punishment. (Reproduced from Kelleher and Morse, 1964.)

biturates release and reinstate punishment-suppressed behavior. This has been demonstrated with the Geller-Seifter procedure (1960), an FR/FR punishment schedule (Fig. 4-2) (Kelleher and Morse, 1964), and a multiple VI/VI punishment schedule (Morse, 1964) (Figs. 3-10 and 3-11). The latter is especially interesting because the stimulation of reinforced and punished behavior was demonstrated simultaneously. Their powerful effect on punishment together with their general facilitatory effect may explain why barbiturates have been used so successfully as minor tranquilizers to treat anxiety states. Indeed, in many studies, barbiturates proved to have a more powerful punishment effect than the bensodiazepines, which were promoted as *specific* anti-anxiety drugs. The dissociation of the effects of amphetamines and barbiturates on punishment suggests that brainstem arousal mechanisms do not underlie this effect. Nor do the depressant effects of barbiturates account for their effects in releasing behavior suppressed by punishment, since 10 mg/kg of pentobarbital, which reinstates punishment-suppressed behavior, also stimulates reinforced behavior. It remains to be seen if tryptaminergic and cholinergic mechanisms of the limbic and hypothalamic systems mediate the anti-anxiety effects, as Stein et al. (1973) have suggested in the case of the benzodiazepines.

EFFECTS OF DRUGS AND HORMONES ON LEARNING AND MEMORY

Introduction

The plasticity of the brain that allows its functions to change adaptively in response to experience is clearly one of the highest functions of the CNS and also one of the least clearly understood at this time. The cellular and biochemical changes associated with learning and memory are largely unknown. Most neurobiologists believe that these phenomena are associated in some way with changes in the connectivity of neurons in the brain, but there is very little clear-cut evidence that such changes occur in any particular learning situation. There have been many attempts by biochemists to explain the processes of learning and memory in simple chemical terms—suggestions, for example, that memory may be associated with the synthesis of specific informational macromolecules in the brain. Such naive hypotheses, however, seem to bear little relation to the real nervous system. A number of claims that "memories" could be transferred from the brains of trained animals to those of untrained animals by means of extracts containing such specific chemical substances as ribonucleic acids, proteins, or peptides have also failed to stand up to the crucial test of reproducibility when examined in other laboratories. The unsatisfactory state of our knowledge in this area does not mean that drug effects on the processes of learning and memory cannot be studied, and, indeed, a large literature exists on such effects. We can only give a highly selective review of some of the psychopharmacological aspects of this problem.

Effects of inhibitors of protein synthesis

Many studies of the effects of drugs that inhibit protein synthesis on learning and memory have been reported. Such drugs are, by their nature, toxic substances, since they can inhibit protein synthesis in all of the tissues of the body. It is impossible, for example, to use such drugs repeatedly at doses sufficiently high to completely inhibit protein synthesis for long periods of time in mammals because of their lethal effects. It is, therefore, important to distinguish any specific effects that these compounds may have on learning and memory from non-specific effects caused simply by their generally toxic action. In properly controlled studies, this distinction can be made by demonstrating that such drugs as CYCLOHEXIMIDE, ACETOXYCYCLOHEXIMIDE, and PUROMYCIN do not impair the acquisition of a learned task, although they are often found to impair the subsequent retention of the mem-

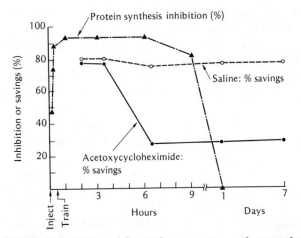

Fig. 4-3 Effect of acetoxycycloheximide on protein synthesis in the brain and on memory. Mice were injected subcutaneously with 240 μg acetoxycycloheximide 30 minutes before training to escape shock by choosing the lighted limb of a T-maze to a criterion of five out of six consecutive correct responses. Different groups were tested for retention (per cent savings) at each of the indicated times. (From Barondes and Cohen, 1967.)

ory of the learning. For example, Barondes and Cohen (1967) showed that acetoxycycloheximide, when given to mice at doses large enough to cause nearly complete inhibition of protein synthesis in the cerebrum, did not prevent the animals from learning a simple positional or light/dark discrimination in a T-maze. Retention of this learning also remained normal for up to 3 hours after the initial acquisition, although retention at 6 hours, 1 day, or 7 days after learning was markedly impaired (Fig. 4-3). These and similar results have suggested that learning itself and the short-term memory that persists for a period of a few hours following training do not depend on ongoing protein synthesis in the brain, whereas the process of consolidation by which short memory is converted into some longer-term storage form may be crucially dependent (in some as yet unknown manner) on cerebral protein synthesis. Inhibitors of protein synthesis, like electroconvulsive shock treatment, can also lead to retrograde amnesia if they are given during this consolidation period, which seems to start during the acquisition itself and continues for some hours thereafter. Thus, in mice or goldfish trained on simple discrimination tasks, electric shock, cycloheximide, or puromycin can prevent long-term memory formation if given immediately after the training period but not if administration is further delayed. In goldfish, the period of susceptibility to protein synthesis inhibitors can be prolonged if the animals are kept in water of 10° C rather than at the normal 20° C, suggesting that the succession from short- to long-term memory storage involves some thermochemical reactions in the CNS. The Flexners (Flexner and Flexner, 1967) found that puromycin induced retrograde amnesia if given by intracerebral injection to mice even several days after the initial training. Cycloheximide, however, did not work in this way, although it is an even more potent inhibitor of protein synthesis. It seems likely that the curious effects of puromycin are due to an induction of abnormal electric activity in the brain by the drug, rather than to an inhibition of protein synthesis.

In conclusion, there seems to be a well-established effect of inhibitors of cerebral protein synthesis in preventing the long-term consolidation of memories. This is not too surprising, since, if such consolidation does involve changes in neuronal connections, presumably some structural changes involving the synthesis of macromolecules will be required at this stage. The effects of protein synthesis inhibitors on memory consolidation, however, have thus far not elucidated the nature of the macromolecules involved in such changes, or their cellular location.

Effects of hormones on learning and memory

There have been many reports in recent years that hormones, particularly of the pituitary-adrenal system, can influence learning and memory in animals. De Wied (1974), for example, has summarized the findings of his group on the remarkable effects of peptide hormones on the acquisition and extinction of conditioned behavior. The peptide hormone ADRENOCORTICOTROPIN (ACTH) is not particularly effective in modifying the acquisition of avoidance behavior or its extinction in normal rats, but its effects are striking in hypophysectomized rats. Such animals, which lack the normal source of ACTH, show an impaired acquisition of avoidance conditioning and an unusually rapid extinction of such behavior once it has been established. Administration of small doses of ACTH to hypophysectomized rats restores normal acquisition and extinction behavior. Furthermore, this effect of ACTH does not appear to be related to the normal endocrine actions of ACTH in promoting steroid secretion from the adrenal gland, since the behavioral effects were elicited by such related hormones as melanocyte-stimulating hormone (MSH), or by fragments of ACTH containing only the seven amino acids at positions 4-10 at the amino terminal end; such molecules are without activity on the adrenals. A series of synthetic peptides similar to the active fragment of the ACTH molecule has been tested; one is devoid of adrenal cortical stimulatory action but is one-thousand times more potent in enhancing acquisition and prolonging extinction of conditioned behavior than the active fragment of ACTH. Injection of nanogram quantities of this substance is sufficient to elicit the behavioral changes. The substance was also active when injected intracerebrally. Such findings are provocative and suggest possible functions for endocrine hormones or related substances in controlling higher neuronal functions; they may perhaps be related in some manner to the over-all role of the pituitary-adrenal system in mediating peripheral and cerebral changes in response to environmental stress.

Many studies have also been made in which steroid hormones of various types were administered by local micro-application directly into various parts of the brain. Often this is done by introducing a very small amount of solid steroid hormone at the end of a fine implanted cannula. The relatively insoluble steroid then slowly diffuses into the surrounding brain tissue, and its effect may persist for many days. Implantation of steroid sex hormones into various brain regions in this way has profound effects on reproductive behavior in both male and female animals. Implants of such glucocorticoid hormones as CORTICOSTERONE or DEXAMETHASONE into various regions in the ascending reticular system or in the limbic forebrain of the rat were found to facilitate extinction of conditioned avoidance behavior—an action opposite to that induced by the ACTH analogues described above. The steroids were effective in facilitating extinction even in hypophysectomized rats, indicating that they did not act simply by inhibiting ACTH release from the pituitary, but rather by some direct cerebral effects.

Effects of other drugs on learning and memory

Cholinergic mechanisms are thought to function in the CNS processes related to learning and memory. In a wide range of species and tasks, the anticholinergics (i.e., drugs that block cholinergic receptors), such as atropine and scopolamine, have been shown to impair learning (Berger and Stein, 1969). The tasks studied include active and passive avoidance, conditioned suppression using shock, habituation to a novel stimulus, and performance on matching to sample of colors. Some theorists (Carlton, 1963) have suggested that the cholinergic system is most important for tasks that involve some kind of behavioral inhibition, i.e., responding under one condition and not under another, as in a go, no-go discrimination task. The generality of this thesis remains to be explored in situations in which responding is eliminated with differential reinforcement, extinction, and punishment.

Atropine and scopolamine themselves have this effect, but

their quaternary nitrogen derivatives, which do not pass the blood-brain barrier, are inactive. Carlton (1963) found that atropine methyl nitrate did not affect avoidance behavior in the rat, and Jarvik and collaborators reported that scopolamine methyl bromide did not impair accuracy of matching to sample in the monkey, although the response rate was depressed on this task. If anticholinergics impair learning, substances that enhance cholinergic activity at the synapse would be expected to enhance acquisition, and, indeed, this is the case. Anticholinesterases, which inhibit the ACh degrading enzyme and thus result in more transmitter being available in the synaptic cleft, are reported to facilitate acquisition of bar-pressing alteration and brightness-detection tasks in rats (Warburton, 1972). On both these tasks, anticholinergics impair learning.

Warburton has tried to characterize the nature of the behavioral change induced by cholinergic manipulations and to identify the neural sites mediating these effects. Using a task in which a change in the intensity of a light indicated that responding is appropriate, he applied signal detection analysis to the behavior and concluded that cholinergic manipulation affected the sensory decisions of the animals rather than their response strategy. Jarvik's observation of impaired accuracy in matching to sample in the absence of response impairment supported this conclusion. Enhanced cholinergic activity appears to improve sensory filtering processes, thereby strengthening the tendency to ignore irrelevant stimuli and improving discrimination. The ascending reticular formation projections to the sensory cortex are likely to be the neural substrate for this cholinergic mechanism. A related cholinergic circuit passing through the hippocampus is also involved in this form of behavioral control.

Not surprisingly, memory is also affected by cholinergic manipulation. Anticholinergics used as pre-anesthetic medication have long been observed to produce amnesia in man. Oliverio (1968) found that scopolamine impaired acquisition and retention of avoidance behavior in the mouse. In an intriguing series of experiments, Deutch (1971) investigated the effect of cholinergic manipulations at various times after the learning experience. He reported that, in undrugged rats, the strength of the memory for simple appetitive or shock avoidance tasks changed over the first 10 days after learning. Immediate retention was excellent but faded by 3 days only to re-emerge strongly at about 10 to 12 days. Deutch saw this as evidence for a biphasic memory consolidation process: an immediate short-term mechanism that is gradually superceded by a more permanent one. Since the pharmacological sensitivity of the brain to cholinergic manipulations mirrors these normal fluctuations in retention performance, he suggests that cholinergic synapses are involved in both processes. Soon after acquisition of learning, cholinergic activity is high but then wanes to re-emerge strongly. Anticholinesterases, such as diisopropylfluorophosphate or physostigmine, if given when cholinergic activity is high, further increase the synaptic availability of ACh to levels that are incompatible with synaptic efficiency, and retention of learning is impaired. If given on day 3, when cholinergic activity is low, however, the cholinergic stimulation produced by these drugs improves retention. By day 10, the drugs again push cholinergic synaptic activity too high. Anticholinergic drugs show a mirror image pattern of anticholinesterases in their effects on retention. When cholinergic activity is high, blockade of some receptors hardly impedes behavior, but, on day 3, when cholinergic activity is low, the block is sufficient to impair behavior.

There is no area in behavior pharmacology more fraught with experimental traps than the study of pharmacologically induced changes in learning and memory. Only the most carefully designed experiments avoid the pitfalls (Weiss and Heller, 1969). Even then the final answer is complicated in the case of cholinergic drugs. In addition to effects on acquisition and retention, the cholinergic drugs alter the habituation response of the animal to the testing environment. Even more importantly, the physiological changes induced peripherally by, for example, injections of the anticholinergics can serve as interoceptive discriminative cues, and ideal conditions for state-dependent learning effects are thus created (Overton, 1966).

There are several reports that, in rats, such excitant drugs as STRYCHNINE, METRAZOL, and MAGNESIUM PEMOLINE improve learning on maze tasks. Strychnine given immediately before trials in a maze speeds acquisition, but the interpretation of these results is compromised by the finding that the same thing happens if the drug is given 3 days before training. Facilitation is also seen if the drug is given immediately after the trials, and this effect does not appear to be due to reinforcement by the drug itself. It is likely that these effects of excitant drugs are non-specific and relate to the general facilitation of neural activity and behavior they induce. Certainly, there are no plausible neurochemical explanations of these effects.

MOOD-MODIFYING DRUGS

Classification and neuropharmacological properties

Introduction and classification

Clinically, depression is characterized by a lowering of mood and is often classified as "endogenous" or "reactive." Endogenous depression often recurs in a regular phasic manner and is not obviously correlated with environmental events; depression of mood alternates with periods of normality in the so-called unipolar depressions. In many cases, abnormal heightening of mood (mania) alternates with the periods of depression in the so-called bipolar or manic-depressive psychoses. The reactive depressions, by contrast, consist of mood abnormalities elicited by stressful environmental events. Depressive psychoses, although they resemble to some degree the mood changes of schizophrenia, are not characterized by the thought disorders, hallucinations, and lack of contact with the real world of schizophrenia.

As with many other classes of psychoactive drugs, the anti-depressants and anti-manic drugs were discovered by accident. During treatment of patients for tuberculosis with the compound IPRONIAZID, it was noticed that this drug had a significant mood-elevating effect. This discovery was followed by the observation that iproniazid is a powerful inhibitor of the enzyme monoamine oxidase (MAO), and this led to the development of a whole family of antidepressant drugs that are MAO inhibitors. A second important series of drugs was discovered when numerous structural analogues of chlorpromazine were synthesized and tested. Replacement of the sulfur atom in the phenothiazine ring of the drug promazine with a methylene bridge gave the compound IMIPRAMINE, which had no neuroleptic properties but was instead found to have an important mood-elevating action. This change from the flat tricyclic phenothiazine structure to a "skewed" three-ring system based on the iminodibenzyl nucleus led to the evolution of another large family of compounds known as the tricyclic antidepressants (Fig. 4-4).

More recently it has been found that the administration of small doses of simple inorganic salts of lithium has an important anti-manic effect in manic-depressive psychoses. An antidepressant effect has also been claimed for lithium salts.

A variety of MAO inhibitors and tricyclics are currently in use as antidepressant drugs. Many of the MAO inhibitors are hydrazine compounds that evolved from iproniazid but are considerably more potent than the parent compound, e.g., PHENIPRAZINE (Catron). Others are non-hydrazines, such as PARGYLINE (Eutonyl) and TRANYLCYPROMINE (Parnate) (see Fig. 2-16). The tricyclics include imipramine (still widely used), its desmethyl derivative DESIPRAMINE, the 3-chloro analogue, CHLORIMIPRA-MINE, and another important series of compounds derived from AMITRIPTYLINE—NORTRIPTYLINE and PROTRIPTYLINE (Fig. 4-4). Imipramine and amitriptyline are metabolized *in vivo* by the liver to give the demethylated derivatives desipramine and nortriptyline (Fig. 4-4), and these are both pharmacologically

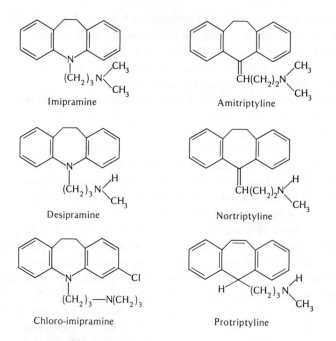

Imipramine

Amitriptyline

Desipramine

Nortriptyline

Chloro-imipramine

Protriptyline

Fig. 4-4 Tricyclic antidepressant drugs.

as active or even more active than the parent compounds. This is thus a good example of drug metabolism giving rise to active products, a process that may be related to the delayed onset and prolonged actions of the parent drugs.

Neuropharmacological properties

The MAO inhibitors, as their name implies, are all powerful inhibitors of monoamine oxidase (MAO) in the brain and in other tissues. All of the compounds in clinical use as antidepressants produce an irreversible inhibition of this enzyme when administered *in vivo,* and their effects are thus very long lasting.

Indeed, recovery of MAO activity in brain and peripheral tissues after treatment with such compounds as pargyline occurs only as new enzyme molecules are synthesized to replace the irreversibly inhibited enzyme. As mentioned in Chapter 2 (p. 112), MAO is involved in the metabolic breakdown of both the catecholamines and 5-HT. After treatment with an MAO inhibitor, there is a rise in the concentration of NE, DA, and especially 5-HT in animal brains, and it is generally assumed that the drugs act to make more of these transmitter amines available for release at adrenergic and tryptaminergic synapses in the brain. There have been, however, no direct demonstrations that this is the case, in either the CNS or the peripheral adrenergic neurons. A rise in the storage level of transmitter need not necessarily mean that more transmitter will be released in response to nerve activity—nevertheless, this remains the most parsimonious explanation of the mode of action of MAO inhibitors.

The idea that MAO inhibitors act by making more catecholamine or 5-HT available at aminergic synapses also fits neatly with the postulated mode of action of the tricyclic antidepressant drugs. These compounds do not inhibit MAO, but they are all potent inhibitors of catecholamine- and 5-HT-uptake mechanisms. Imipramine, amitriptyline, and, especially, their desmethyl analogues are among the most potent inhibitors of the NE uptake system in noradrenergic neurons known (see Chapter 2, p. 114). They are effective in *in vitro* experiments at concentrations as low as 10^{-8}M (the equivalent of only a few picograms of drug per milliliter). The same drugs, however, are also very potent inhibitors of the 5-HT uptake system associated with 5-HT-containing neurons in the CNS. There is a somewhat different structure-activity relationship for inhibition of 5-HT and NE uptake by the tricyclics (Table 4-2), desipramine being the most potent inhibitor of NE uptake and chlorimipramine the most potent inhibitor of 5-HT uptake. Nevertheless, since the clinically used drugs are moderately potent inhibitors of both systems, it is impossible to say whether the action on one or the

TABLE 4-2

INHIBITION OF AMINE UPTAKE BY TRICYCLICS

Amine	IC_{50}* (μM)		
	5-HT	NE	DA
Chlorimipramine	0.04	0.30	–
Imipramine	0.50	0.20	8.70
Desipramine	2.50	0.03	50.00

* IC_{50} values (drug concentration needed to cause 50% inhibition of amine uptake) were determined in rat brain synaptosome preparations (L. L. Iversen, 1974).

other amine system is the more important. The tricyclic antidepressants are, however, very much less active as inhibitors of DA uptake in dopaminergic neurons, so this seems to be ruled out as a site of action. At synapses using NE or 5-HT as transmitters, the tricyclic antidepressant drugs would be expected to enhance and potentiate the effects of the released transmitter by preventing the normally rapid removal of released amine by tissue uptake mechanisms. In peripheral adrenergic systems, this is exactly the effect observed; drugs such as imipramine or desipramine markedly potentiate the responses of smooth muscle tissues to sympathetic nerve stimulation or to applied NE.

It seems likely, therefore, that antidepressant drugs owe their action to a potentiation of NE and/or 5-HT at synapses in the CNS. This hypothesis is supported also by the behavioral effects of these drugs, particularly their ability to antagonize or counteract behavioral depression induced by reserpine or tetrabenazine, which act in the opposite manner to reduce the availability of catecholamines and 5-HT in the brain. It should be remembered, however, that we do not know whether the effect on NE or on 5-HT is the most important in explaining the mood-elevating effects of these drugs. Indeed it is quite possible that such effects are related to neither compound. The MAO inhibitors, for example, lead to increased concentrations in the brain of a variety of aromatic amines that are usually present only in minute amounts; these include the phenylethylamine derivatives, tyramine, phenylethanolamine, and octopamine, and the indolamine, tryptamine. The accumulation of such amines might well have important neuropharmacological consequences, although they are not yet understood. The accumulation of such amines as tyramine after MAO inhibition is probably related to the inhibition of MAO in the liver and intestine by MAO inhibitors. The enzyme is very abundant in these peripheral tissues, where it normally plays an important role in destroying and rendering harmless such pharmacologically active amines as tyramine; these amines are present in substantial amounts in many foods of plant origin and are absorbed in quite large quantities from the diet. Because this detoxification mechanism is abolished after MAO inhibition, ingestion of foods rich in these amines, such as certain cheeses and wines, can have undesirable and even fatal consequences in patients being treated with such drugs. A sudden absorption of a large dose of tyramine can lead to serious cardiovascular disturbances, since this amine stimulates the entire cardiovascular system by promoting a release of NE, which it displaces from sympathetic nerve terminals. For this reason, patients treated with MAO inhibitors must observe strict dietary precautions; the potential toxicity of the MAO inhibitors has led to their gradual replacement in clinical use by the tricyclic antidepressant drugs, which do not produce these undesirable side effects.

The inorganic salts of lithium have a variety of effects on excitable tissue. Lithium ions can replace sodium in the generation of the nerve action potential, but, unlike sodium, lithium is not rapidly pumped out of cells by the active pump mechanism; it tends, therefore, to accumulate, rendering the tissue less readily excitable. The precise mode of action of the antimanic actions of lithium salts, however, is not known.

Behavioral pharmacology of antidepressants

Tricyclic compounds

The behavioral effects of the tricyclic antidepressants are extremely difficult to characterize and dissociate from those of the neuroleptic phenothiazines. This should perhaps not be surprising in view of their chemical similarity and their shared efficacy in modulating affect and mood. When relatively large doses are given, both have a sedative effect on spontaneous motor behavior, although motor depression after imipramine is not associated with catatonia. Imipramine produces dose-dependent decrements in responding on FR schedules for food reinforcement. FI responding is also depressed, and the scalloped pattern of responding is reduced to a low regular pattern throughout the interval. Responding maintained by shock-escape or shock avoidance is affected in a similar manner (Cook and Kelleher, 1962).

There are reports, as with chlorpromazine, that in conditioned avoidance situations, where both avoidance and escape can be evaluated, imipramine will abolish the avoidance response, leaving the escape response intact.

A change in the power of environmental stimuli to control behavior is cited as an explanation for this and related results. This is supported by the finding that avoidance under certain conditions is not impaired by either chlorpromazine or imipramine. Cook and Kelleher describe a concurrent schedule for the squirrel monkey in which shock is avoided on a non-discriminated Sidman schedule, and every 100th response is reinforced with food. The low avoidance rate after each reinforcement is not affected by imipramine, although the high rate of responding just before each reinforcement is depressed.

The same authors also investigated imipramine on their two-key paradigm, where presses on one key produced reinforcement and presses on the other discriminative stimuli (S^D or S^Δ), indicating whether or not reinforcement was available on the other key. In the pigeon, imipramine, like chlorpromazine, increased responding to the "discrimination" key, and it was concluded that "imipramine and chlorpromazine have some common pharmacological properties."

It has also been stated, as with chlorpromazine, that negatively reinforced behavior is more sensitive to the disruptive effects of imipramine than is positively reinforced behavior. Cook and Kelleher (1962) describe a concurrent avoidance FR 100 schedule, where the high rates of FR responding were affected at doses of imipramine that did not interfere with Sidman avoidance. Weissman (1959) used a four-segment schedule, time out–Sidman avoidance–continuous reinforcement –time out, and reported that avoidance was depressed before responding on the continuous reinforcement schedule. But these interpretations must be accepted with caution. The results purport to show a greater sensitivity of shock-reinforced behavior to antidepressants, but they should be examined in the way Dews and Morse evaluated the reports of a similar effect for chlorpromazine (see p. 249). The soundest approach to this problem is to *equate* the base-line behaviors controlled by shock and food. This has been achieved by Kelleher and Morse (1964) in the squirrel monkey, using either FI shock-escape or FI food reinforcement schedules. In this case, imipramine produces an identical dose-dependent depression of both behavioral base lines. Different monkeys were trained on the two schedules, and it remains to be shown on an alternating FI escape FI food schedule that the same results would be found. If imipramine has any selective effect on negatively reinforced behavior, it has yet to be clearly defined.

Vaillant (1964) reports one of the few efforts to quantitatively dissociate the behavioral effects of imipramine and chlorpromazine. The pigeon is the only species in which both chlorpromazine and imipramine have been found to increase rates of responding on food reinforcement schedules. Valiant used a two-key situation; on the blue key, an FR 30 was programmed for six reinforcements and then, on the red key, FI 5 minutes was programmed for six reinforcements. Both key lights remained on throughout the session, and reinforcement was available alternately for the two keys. In these circumstances, birds distributed behavior between the keys; typical scalloped patterns of responding during the FI program were interspersed with bursts of responding to the FR key. During the FR programs, the typical high rate of FR responding occurred, but there were no responses on the FI key. Imipramine increased the rates of responding on both keys without interfering with the control that the schedule and discriminative stimuli had over the behavior (Fig. 4-5 A-C). By contrast, during the FI phase of the schedule, chlorpromazine depressed FI responding (Fig. 4-5C), while increasing unreinforced responding on the FR key (Fig. 4-5B). Unfortunately, a complex behavioral method of this kind is not a very useful tool for evaluating tricyclic antidepressants. Furthermore, the rate-increasing effects of antidepressants are seen only in the pigeon. In the search for behavioral methods of characterizing antidepressants, various indirect methods have been investigated. First, tricyclic antidepressants have been found to potentiate the behavioral effects of amphetamine. Stein, for example, reported such a potentiation of amphetamine-induced increases in the rate of intracranial self-stimulation in rats with implanted stimulating electrodes. Several authors have demonstrated a potentiation of amphetamine-induced locomotor activity in the rat. This effect has now been shown to be due to the fact that the tricyclic antidepressants impede the enzymatic degradation of amphetamine. The effect is species-specific and is not found, for example, in the mouse.

Second, and again unlike chlorpromazine, the tricyclics antagonize the depressant effects of reserpine and tetrabenazine in some species. McKearney (1968b) has shown that, in the rat,

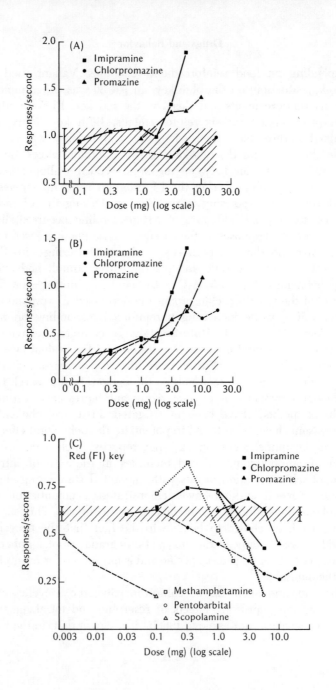

imipramine does *not* antagonize the depressant effects of tetrabenazine on operant responding. Antagonism is seen in the pigeon, but, as McKearney points out, this is a species in which imipramine alone has marked rate-increasing effects. It is one of the enigmas and frustrations of behavioral pharmacology that an animal behavioral model of depression has not yet been developed. Animals show states akin to depression when a mate or infant is lost, as Goodall describes from her observation of chimpanzees, but it seems to be a difficult condition to induce experimentally. Baltzer and Weiskrantz (1970)

Fig. 4-5 (A) Dose-effect curves for the effects of chlorpromazine, imipramine, and promazine, on the total responding of pigeons during the FI phase of a two-key concurrent; mix FR 30, ext; mix ext, FI 300 seconds. The rate in responses per second indicates the average over-all rate on both keys. All points represent averaged duplicate determinations for four birds except that the control value (X) is the average for eight control sessions for each bird. The hatched area indicates a range of two standard errors of the mean control rate. The asterisk indicates a significant elevation of rate at an 0.05 level of confidence (Student's t-test). (B) Dose-response curves for the effects of imipramine, chlorpromazine, and promazine on the behavior of pigeons during FI on the blue (FR) key. The hatched area indicates a range of two standard errors of the mean control rate. All drug points represent average duplicate determinants for four birds. (C) Comparative dose-response curves for several drugs on rate of responding on the red (FI) key during the entire FI phase. The two lowest doses of chlorpromazine and the points for scopolamine, pentobarbital, and methamphetamine represent averaged single determinations of four birds. Due to their shorter duration of action, methamphetamine and pentobarbital were given 15 minutes before the run, and the experiment was run for only two instead of three FR-FI cycles. This schedule change led to somewhat higher control rates on the red (FI) key. The asterisk indicates that elevation of rate is statistically significant ($p < .01$) by the Student's t-test. The apparent elevation of FI rate by the lowest doses of pentobarbital and methamphetamine was not significantly different from control rates for the 3 weeks during which these values were obtained. X indicates the averaged rate of six control sessions for each bird obtained over a 6-month period. The hatched area represents a range of two standard errors of the mean control rate. (Reproduced from Vaillant, 1964.)

hope that the "elation" test described earlier (Chapter 1, pp. 53-54) may be a useful model for testing antidepressants.

MAO inhibitors

Behavioral studies of the MAO inhibitors have been closely correlated with neuropharmacological studies of these compounds. The inhibition of MAO results in an accumulation of amine transmitters in the brain, and behavioral correlates of these neuropharmacological changes have been sought. Since MAO inhibition affects the synaptic availability of DA, NE, and 5-HT, it has been difficult to correlate any behavioral change with any particular amine. A slow increase in spontaneous activity has been reported, which corresponds in its time-course to the increase in amine levels after certain MAO inhibitors. Because of their chemical structural similarity to amphetamine, some MAO inhibitors have additional stimulant properties and can induce a faster increase in spontaneous locomotor activity.

ICS is one behavioral measure that has yielded positive effects with antidepressants. The tricyclics potentiate amphetamine-induced intracranial stimulation (ICS) by increasing brain amphetamine levels. The MAO inhibitors, however, increase ICS behavior directly, which may well relate to their own effect on amine systems. Poschel and Ninteman (1963) reported that 100 mg/kg iproniazid increased ICS, markedly, after the second dose. Tranylcypromine at doses that do not affect locomotor activity prevents the normal abolishment of ICS responding by tetrabenazine.

MAO inhibitors will also reverse tetrabenazine-induced depression of shock-avoidance behavior in the rat. On this parameter they again differ from the tricyclics (Fig. 4-6).

Stein and Wise (1969) suggest that ICS reflects activity in reward systems in the hypothalamus/limbic areas, and it has also been suggested that depression could reflect sluggishness in such systems, which can be reversed with drugs that increase the synaptic availability of amines. If this is the case, it is surprising that tricyclics, which also increase synaptic amines by blocking re-uptake, have no such effect on ICS behavior.

Lithium

In 1963, Danish workers (Schou, 1963) reported that lithium carbonate was a useful drug for treating and preventing the manic phases of cyclical depression. This was a very useful finding for, although the tricyclics and MAO inhibitors were in successful use for treating depressive phases, the manic phase was unresponsive to these drugs and to the phenothiazines.

At this time, despite its increasing use, the neuropharmacological basis of lithium's effect remains obscure, and study of its behavioral effects in animal model systems has hardly begun.

OPIATES

Classification and neuropharmacological properties

The group of drugs known as the "opiates" or sometimes as the "narcotics" comprises the various naturally occurring alkaloids of the opium poppy, of which MORPHINE is the main example, and various synthetic drugs with similar actions. The compounds most extensively studied are morphine and its diacetyl derivative HEROIN and the synthetic compounds LEVORPHANOL, MEPERIDINE, and METHADONE (Fig. 4-7).

The opiates have a complex neuropharmacological action; they are extremely useful drugs clinically for the alleviation of severe pain (analgesia). Their analgesic action, however, is also associated with complex psychological effects, of which their ability to induce a state of euphoria is the main reason for their importance as drugs of abuse. The particular state of well-being induced by the opiates defies description; after intravenous administration, these drugs lead to immediate physical sensations that are extremely pleasurable. The marked tendency of re-

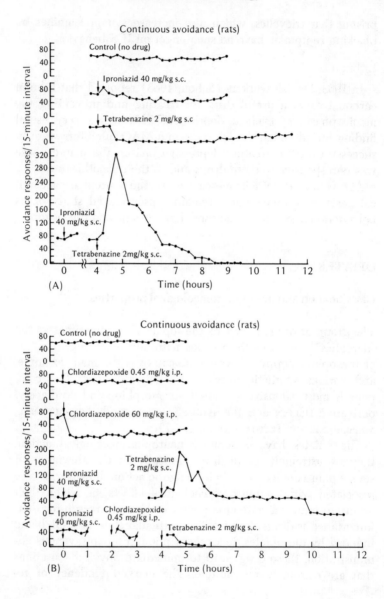

peated drug administration to lead to tolerance and physical dependence, however, makes them dangerous drugs of addiction.

For many years an intensive search has been made for safer analgesic drugs with the pain-relieving properties of morphine but without the addictive and psychotropic properties of the parent drug. Although many synthetic opiates have been discovered—for example, levorphanol, meperidine, pethidine, and methadone—none of them differs basically from morphine in addiction potential. Methadone has been used increasingly in the treatment of morphine and heroin addicts largely because its action is of longer duration than morphine, and the withdrawal syndrome is less severe.

An important discovery, however, has been that some drugs, such as NALORPHINE and CYCLAZOCINE (Fig. 4-7), are potent analgesics although they appear to act as morphine antagonists with regard to the psychotropic effects of morphine (Weiss, 1956). Such morphine antagonists can precipitate a withdrawal syndrome in addicts or in animals chronically treated with morphine, although in normal animals they have few or no obvious behavioral effects. These antagonists may represent the first success in dissociating the analgesic action of the opiates from their

---

Fig. 4-6 (A) Effects of iproniazid, tetrabenazine, and the combination on rate of lever pressing of rats in the continuous avoidance procedure. *First record:* avoidance response rate during a 5-hour control session; *second record:* iproniazid alone had no significant effect on behavior; *third record:* tetrabenazine alone produced a nearly complete loss of responding; *fourth record:* in rats pretreated with iproniazid, tetrabenazine produced marked stimulation shown by the increased rate of lever pressing. (B) Effect of chlordiazepoxide on the stimulation induced by iproniazid and tetrabenazine. *First record:* Control behavior; *second record:* a small dose of chlordiazepoxide had no effect on normal avoidance behavior; *third record:* it was necessary to increase the dose of chlordiazepoxide to 60 mg/kg to markedly suppress normal avoidance behavior; *fourth record:* stimulation produced by iproniazid and tetrabenazine ʻ(cf. Fig. 4-3); *fifth record:* administration of a small dose of chlordiazepoxide 2 hours prior to tetrabenazine, in rats pretreated with iproniazid, completely blocked the stimulation. (Reproduced from Zbinden and Randall, 1967.)

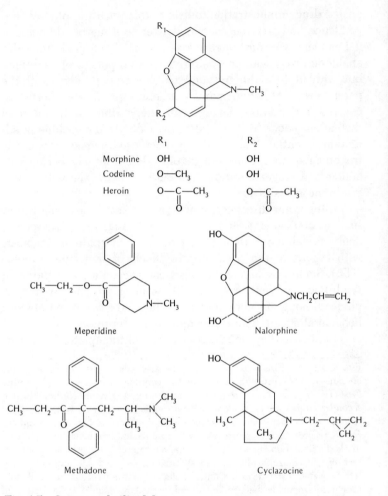

Fig. 4-7 Opiates and related drugs.

other less desirable effects. Unfortunately, these drugs have not proved suitable for clinical use as analgesics because they tend to have such unpleasant side effects as hallucinations and psychosis-like states.

An important step forward in understanding the basic mechanism of action of morphine has been achieved very recently by the establishment of an *in vitro* biochemical system in which opiate agonists and antagonists can be studied. This system can measure the specific binding of radioactively labeled opiate drugs to their receptor sites in brain homogenates, and it has already allowed precise comparisons of the potencies of many agonist and antagonist drugs and a mapping of the distribution of opiate receptor sites in various brain regions to be made. The receptor sites may also be identified ultimately in this way and their normal pharmacological function determined. The receptors appear to be most concentrated in the amygdala and in periventricular gray matter in the brain stem of the monkey brain (Kuhar et al., 1973).

Tolerance and dependence

The opiates are the drugs *par excellence* for illustrating the phenomena of tolerance and dependence. Tolerance is readily induced in man or animals by repeated drug administration (see Fig. 2-4). After some weeks of drug administration, the animal or addict may require twenty to forty times the dose of drug initially used to obtain a given effect. Animals can be trained to self-administer opiate drugs, and the dose of drug administered in this way shows a progressive increase as tolerance develops. Tolerance cannot be explained simply in terms of an increased rate of drug metabolism after chronic use, although this may play some role in the over-all process. The development of "cellular tolerance," of unknown mechanism, seems to be far more important, however (see Chapter 2, p. 76). Cross-tolerance is seen among all the opiate agonists described above.

Physical dependence invariably accompanies the development of tolerance to the opiates. Thus, addicts or chronically treated animals may appear superficially normal in their overt behavior, but a withdrawal syndrome is easily precipitated by stopping drug treatment or more immediately by the administration of an opiate antagonist drug such as NALOXONE. The withdrawal syn-

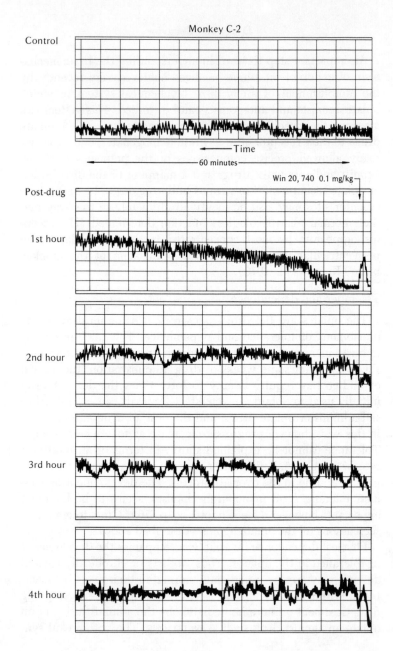

Monkey C-2

Control

←—Time

←——————— 60 minutes ———————→

Win 20, 740 0.1 mg/kg

Post-drug

1st hour

2nd hour

3rd hour

4th hour

210

drome is a complex process with many different components; in man, these include restlessness, craving for the drug, perspiration, chills, fever, vomiting, panting, insomnia, and hyperactivity of the sympathetic system (dilated pupils, piloerection, and hypertension). The withdrawal syndrome can be reversed immediately by administration of morphine or any other opiate agonist drug. The rapid effects of opiate agonists and antagonists in reversing or precipitating withdrawal symptoms strongly suggest that after tolerance has developed a continued occupation of receptor sites by an opiate agonist drug is needed to prevent the onset of withdrawal.

Many theories of the cellular basis for tolerance and dependence have been proposed. It seems likely that some long-term changes take place in the synthesis of macromolecules involved in the action of the drugs. Studies with radiolabeled receptor-binding drugs have so far failed to reveal any long-term change in the number of opiate receptor sites in brain tissue from tolerant animals, however, so some other type of molecule appears to be involved.

Behavioral effects

Morphine

The mood-changing properties of morphine and heroin form only part of a complex profile of psychological and physiological effects induced by these drugs.

Morphine, despite undesirable autonomic side effects, is used clinically as an analgesic, yet the nature of this analgesia and its relationship to its effects on other behaviors remains obscure.

Fig. 4-8 Recording attenuator record of the response of one monkey to 0.1 mg/kg of WIN 20,740. Each segment represents 1 hour; the control segment is the last hour of the 2-hour predrug sample. Time reads from right to left; maximum shock is represented by the top of the record. Each 1-hour segment begins with the shock level reset to zero. (Reproduced from Weiss and Laties, 1964b.)

Behavioral Pharmacology

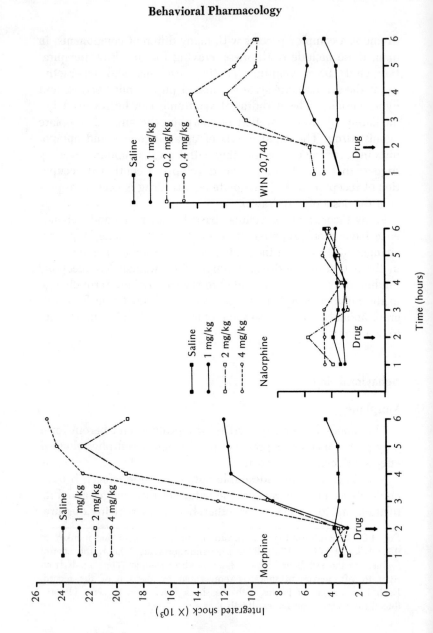

The hot plate test and the tail-flick technique of D'Amour-Smith have been used traditionally for assessing analgesics. But the analgesic action of morphine, nalorphine, and the benzomorphan compounds was most elegantly demonstrated by Weiss and Laties (1964b) who, using electric shocks of variable intensity, titrated the maximum shock level monkeys would tolerate. Monkeys sat in a restraining chair and were shocked through shoes on the feet. The apparatus was programmed so that the animal received a shock of increasing intensity ($<$ 5 ma) every 2 seconds. A lever press between shocks prevented this increase. Thus, by pressing regularly the animal could "hold" the shock at a low level of intensity. Six-hour sessions were given. After a 2-hour control run, morphine or a related compound was injected, and the shock threshold plotted for a further 4 hours. The shock was controlled by a recording attenuator, an apparatus that systematically changes the intensity of a stimulus and plots out its value on a continuous paper record. Both morphine and the benzomorphan (WIN 20, 740) (Fig. 4-8) increased the level of shock monkeys would tolerate; 4 mg/kg of morphine raised the shock level to nearly its maximum (Fig. 4-9). It is tempting to think that this marked change in threshold to painful stimuli underlies the effect of morphine in reducing anxiety associated with pain when used clinically. When morphine was studied on one of the classical behavioral tests for assessing anti-anxiety drugs in animals, however, the results did not support the contention that there is such a relationship between analgesia and mood. On the Geller procedure, rats are reinforced and simultaneously punished with electric shock for lever pressing. Minor tranquilizers (benzodiazepines and barbiturates) produce a marked release from the suppressive effects of punishment, but morphine in doses of 4 mg/kg was quite ineffective, despite the fact that this dose must clearly have been

Fig. 4-9 Hour-by-hour changes in tolerated shock level; the values shown represent mean integrated shock ($N = 5$). (Reproduced from Weiss and Laties, 1964b.)

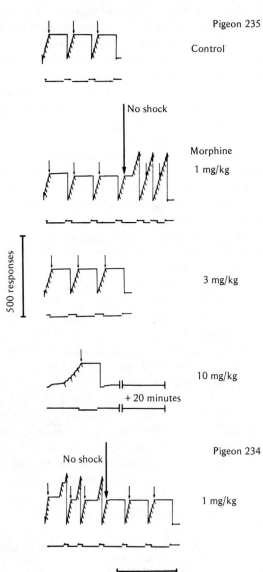

analgesic (Geller et al., 1963). Kelleher and Morse (1964) also failed to reinstate punished responding with morphine in the pigeon (Fig. 4-10). They found that after the punishing electric shock was actually switched off, responding was reinstated much less quickly (Fig. 4-11) than after benzodiazepines and barbiturates (Fig. 4-2), and it may be that the control mediated by their particular procedure is also independent of the painful nature of the suppressive stimulus. This lack of effect of morphine on punished behavior seemed well established until very recently. McMillan (1973a) found that under certain conditions morphine would reinstate punished responding in the pigeon. This result was obtained using a multiple FI/FI punishment schedule, with every response during the punishment component being followed by a 2.5 to 5.2-ma shock of 50-msec duration. Morphine in 0.3 and 1.0 mg/kg amounts restored responding during the punishment component to the same degree as did the benzodiazepines. This result is consonant with the anti-anxiety effect of morphine noted in man. The failure to obtain this result in earlier experiments is difficult to explain. There are, however, differences in species, schedule, and shock parameter between the three studies. On the Geller procedure, with rats, every response was both rewarded and punished during the punishment component, but the shock level was low,

---

Fig. 4-10   Effect of morphine on behavior suppressed by punishment. The first four frames show performance of pigeon 235 on the fixed-ratio procedure in which nonpunishment and punishment components alternated. Shocks were scheduled in punishment components except where indicated. *First record:* control performance; *second record* (start): performance on the same procedure following the intramuscular injection of morphine (1 mg/kg); at the large arrow, scheduled shocks were omitted; *third and fourth records:* the effects of larger doses of morphine—20 minutes in which no responses occurred have been omitted from the 10 mg/kg record; *fifth record:* the effect of morphine on the performance of pigeon 234. Scheduled shocks were omitted at the beginning of the record and then reinstated at the larger arrow. Note that morphine did not prevent the almost immediate return of suppression by punishment with electric shocks. (Reproduced from Kelleher and Morse, 1964.)

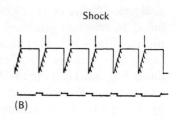

Shock   No shock

(A)

Shock

(B)

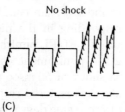

No shock

(C)

No shock

(D)

500 responses

No shock

(E)

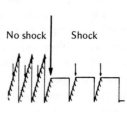

No shock   Shock

(F)

Shock

(G)

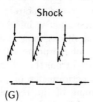

No shock

(H)

10 minutes

0.75 ma. Kelleher and Morse (1964) used high shock levels but punished only the first ten responses of each rewarded FR 30 in the punishment component of their schedule. McMillan (1973a) also punished with a high shock every response made during a rewarded 5-minute FI. This punishment-releasing effect of morphine is clearly an important finding, and the discrepancy between these studies is worth further investigation, especially in view of the fact that McMillan (1973b) reports that on a FR 30, F 15 schedule, with every response in both components punished, morphine failed to reverse suppression.

In common with other CNS sedatives and hypnotics, small doses of morphine stimulate behavior. For example, locomotor activity is stimulated in rodents, and Goldstein and Sheehan (1969) have used this simple behavioral response as an elegant model system for quantifying tolerance to morphine and its analogues. A single dose of 20 mg/kg of levorphanol induces a "running fit" in mice, and, if this dose is repeated every 8 hours, tolerance develops rapidly (Fig. 4-12). The running fit meets the essential criteria for a typical effect of the opioid narcotics. It shows the same high degree of specificity, levorphanol being active whereas the stereoisomer dextrorphan is inactive: the slopes of the dose-response curves are the same for the running

---

Fig. 4-11 The effects of omitting and reinstating scheduled electric shocks on behavior suppresed by punishment. In nonpunishment components, a 30-response, fixed-ratio schedule of food reinforcement was in effect in the presence of an orange stimulus; nonpunishment components terminated after five reinforcements as indicated by the small arrows. In punishment components, a 30-response, fixed-ratio schedule was in effect in the presence of a white stimulus; each of the first ten responses of each ratio produced a brief electric shock. Punishment components terminated after five reinforcements or 3 minutes, as indicated by the resetting of the pen to the bottom of the record. The frames show successive daily sessions except between B and C, where one session is omitted, and between F and G, where two sessions are omitted. The periods during which scheduled shocks were omitted are indicated. Note the records (frames C, D, and H), showing suppression of responding at the beginning of sessions in which scheduled shocks were omitted (spontaneous retrogression). (Reproduced from Kelleher and Morse, 1964.)

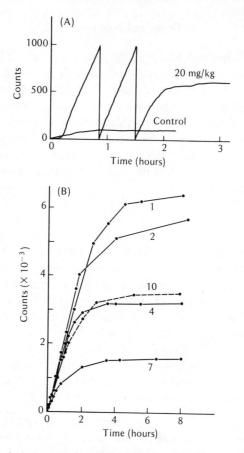

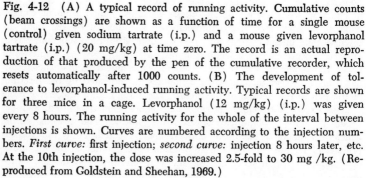

Fig. 4-12 (A) A typical record of running activity. Cumulative counts (beam crossings) are shown as a function of time for a single mouse (control) given sodium tartrate (i.p.) and a mouse given levorphanol tartrate (i.p.) (20 mg/kg) at time zero. The record is an actual reproduction of that produced by the pen of the cumulative recorder, which resets automatically after 1000 counts. (B) The development of tolerance to levorphanol-induced running activity. Typical records are shown for three mice in a cage. Levorphanol (12 mg/kg) (i.p.) was given every 8 hours. The running activity for the whole of the interval between injections is shown. Curves are numbered according to the injection numbers. *First curve:* first injection; *second curve:* injection 8 hours later, etc. At the 10th injection, the dose was increased 2.5-fold to 30 mg /kg. (Reproduced from Goldstein and Sheehan, 1969.)

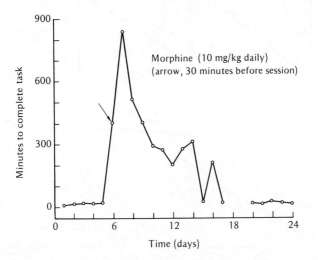

Fig. 4-13 The development of tolerance to the effects of 10 mg/kg of morphine daily on schedule-controlled performance in the pigeon. *Abscissa:* daily sessions; *ordinate:* time to complete the four schedule components composing the daily session. The first five points show the control performance. From the 6th session (arrow), 10 mg/kg of morphine were given 30 minutes before the session. The time to complete the session increased greatly and then gradually returned to control values. The pigeon was injected but not tested on days 18 and 19. (Reproduced from McMillan and Morse, 1967.)

fit and analgesia parameters, and the potency ratio of levorphanol to morphine is 5.0 for both. Nalorphine terminates the running fit, and there is cross-tolerance to morphine.

By contrast, larger doses lead to depression of behavior, as has been observed by Verhave et al. (1959) in rats trained in an avoidance task. The conditioned-avoidance response was lost with a dose of 4 mg/kg, but escape was less affected. In dogs, however, Domino et al. (1958) did not find a loss of shock avoidance except at doses that produce motor deficits and, at this level, escape behavior was more affected than avoidance.

McMillan and Morse (1967) have studied the depressant ef-

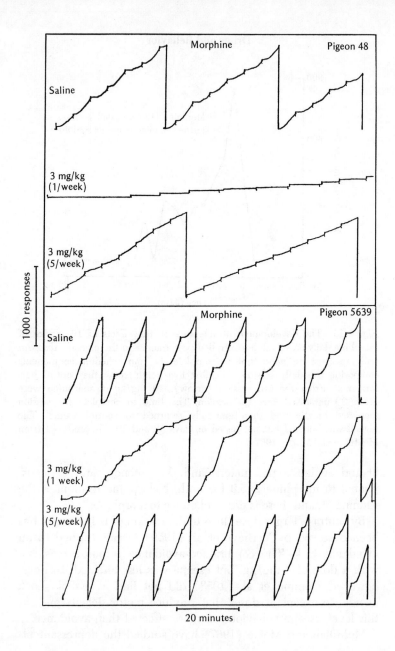

fect of morphine on food-reinforced responding in the pigeons, and these effects, like the excitatory effects, show tolerance after daily injections (Fig. 4-13). When tolerance has developed, the same dose will frequently stimulate response rates rather than depress them (Fig. 4-14). Stimulatory effects of morphine have been seen in man where convulsions eventually occur, but this occurs at doses well above those used for analgesia and therefore cannot be compared to the stimulatory effects seen in rodents with low doses. Spontaneous behavior in the rat is also depressed by larger doses of morphine, but, if these are repeated, tolerance to this effect develops, and the drug induces a highly characteristic form of stereotyped behavior. In rats, this stereotypy is easily distinguished from that produced by larger doses of amphetamine (Schiørring and Hecht, 1974).

It is interesting to speculate as to why some psychoactive drugs are highly addictive, whereas others are not. Both antidepressants and opiates produce elevation of mood, but only the latter are addictive. It is unlikely that all addictive drugs are addictive for the same reason, but, at least, in the case of opiates, Schuster and Woods have produced experimental support for the suggestion of Wikler (1965) that addiction, like withdrawal, may be associated with classical conditioning of environmental stimuli to the physiological effects of the injected drug.

Wikler had suggested that, in opiate dependence, stimuli associated with withdrawal could eventually elicit withdrawal. Goldberg and Schuster (1967) made monkeys dependent on morphine. They were trained to work for food on a schedule of reinforcement, and, when nalorphine was given to the morphine-dependent monkeys, withdrawal occurred and responding

Fig. 4-14 The development of tolerance to the effects of 3 mg/kg of morphine on schedule-controlled performance in the pigeon. Cumulative response records under multiple FR 30 FI 5, pigeons 48 and 5639. The records show the effect of saline, 3 mg/kg of morphine during the first 1/week series, and 3 mg/kg of morphine during the daily morphine series. (Reproduced from McMillan and Morse, 1967.)

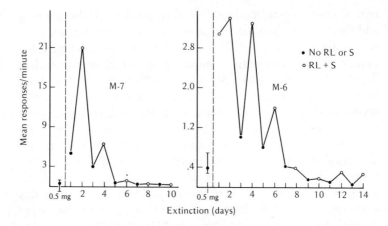

Fig. 4-15   Responses of two monkeys during morphine extinction sessions. On each graph the far left point is the final 5-day average of response rate for morphine reinforcement. To the right of the dashed line, points show extinction data—solid points, absence of response consequence (i.e., no morphine or conditioned stimuli); open circles, response consequence of saline plus red light. Absolute response rates differ in the two animals, but in both the presence of conditioned stimuli increases extinction responding. (Reproduced from Schuster and Woods, 1968.)

for food was depressed. Then a buzzer was sounded during the withdrawal induced by nalorphine, and, after such conditioning, presentation of the buzzer alone induced withdrawal symptoms and depression of bar pressing.

In following up these studies, Schuster and Woods (1968) found that sensory stimuli associated with opiate administration itself could also be conditioned. The monkeys worked on a 6-hour multiple schedule, which started with a 2-hour time-out when no food or drug was available; during 1 hour, in the presence of a green light, food reinforcement was available; and this was followed by 1 hour of white light, with infusion of morphine every 2.5 minutes in the presence of a red light. The 5th hour was the food schedule and the 6th hour a time-out.

After 60 days of drug infusion, the animals were put into morphine extinction. On alternate days, during the 4th hour, the red light without morphine was presented, or the red light was presented, and saline infusion was given. Under the latter condition, an increase in responding was seen in the presence of the red light plus the physical manipulations associated with placebo injection (Fig. 4-15). Since the red light alone did not have this affect, it is suggested that the stimuli associated with the injection had acquired secondary reinforcing properties because of their earlier association with morphine infusion. These are most important observations for understanding the behavioral basis of morphine addiction.

MINOR TRANQUILIZERS

Classification and neuropharmacological properties

The minor tranquilizers are used for treating neurotic as opposed to psychotic symptoms. Neuroses are varied but are generally characterized by anxiety and tension. A variety of pharmacological agents have been used over the years—alcohol being perhaps the most common.

Barbiturates in small doses have been used extensively for their anti-anxiety effect. Their use for this purpose is now out of favor because of the problems of tolerance and dependence and the possible hazards of accidental overdose or suicide associated with the regular prescribing of such drugs to anxious and depressed patients. Nevertheless, as we shall see, barbiturates share the specific attributes of the more potent minor tranquilizers, meprobamate and the more recently discovered benzodiazepines.

When meprobamate was first described, its behavioral effects appeared to be similar to but less dramatic than those of chlorpromazine. The term "minor tranquilizer" came into use to differentiate such drugs from the "major" neuroleptic tranquilizers. In their 1963 review, Cook and Kelleher state that meprobamate

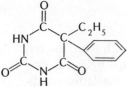

Phenobarbital

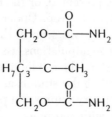

Meprobamate
(Miltown, Equanil)

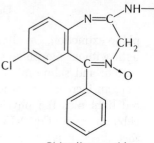

Chlordiazepoxide
(Librium)

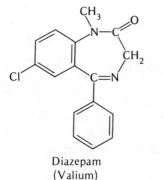

Diazepam
(Valium)

Flurazepam
(Dalmane)

Fig. 4-16 The minor tranquilizers.

and chlordiazepoxide (Librium) "are prescribed for mild behavior disorders." It is interesting to note the progress that has
been made in 10 years. Now that the major and minor tranquilizers have been studied in a wider range of behavioral situations, it is apparent that the differences between them are quali-
tative rather than quantitative. It is for this reason that we
prefer to use the terms "antipsychotics" or "neuroleptics" and
"minor tranquilizers" in this book rather than the traditional
major/minor tranquilizer terminology.

In recent years, the benzodiazepines, exemplified by CHLOR-
DIAZEPOXIDE (LIBRIUM) and DIAZEPAM (VALIUM) (Fig. 4-16),

have found great favor because they combine specific calming and anti-anxiety effects with very low toxicity, so that there is little danger of the accidental or intentional overdose that so frequently occurs with the barbiturates. A large number of related benzodiazepine derivatives have been synthesized and tested, and several of these compounds have proved clinically useful, for example, FLURAZEPAM and NITRAZEPAM (MOGODON). The latter compound is a more powerful hypnotic than is chlordiazepoxide or diazepam and is used to induce sleep rather than to tranquilize.

Very little is known of the neuropharmacological actions of any of these compounds. It has been observed that both the benzodiazepines and the barbiturates reduce the normal rate of turnover of NE, DA, and 5-HT in animal brain. It has been suggested by Stein et al. (1973) that the action of such compounds in slowing 5-HT turnover may be a key point in any explanation of their actions. Stein suggests that 5-HT may act as the transmitter in an ascending system of neurons associated with punishment and that the minor tranquilizers may act to diminish activity in this system of neurons. The drugs do not, however, appear to directly affect monoamine-containing neurons, but presumably act indirectly by affecting some other neuronal system that determines the state of activity of the monoaminergic neurons.

Behavioral pharmacology

Meprobamate

The tranquilizing effect of meprobamate was originally detected when it was observed that it could "tame" monkeys. In doses of 250-400 mg/kg, the drug makes normally truculent monkeys easy to handle, and they do not respond aggressively to man. Although tranquilized, the animals remain responsive to the environment; this taming effect contrasts with the equally potent effect of chlorpromazine in this respect, which leaves the animal withdrawn from the environment. Experimentally induced aggression is also attenuated by meprobamate. Surgical lesions of the septum result in marked aggression in certain species, such as the rat, and meprobamate in doses of 240 mg/kg abolishes this aggression. Chlorpromazine will also sedate such animals, but they become vicious if aroused. If isolated in individual cages for 2 to 3 weeks, mice show attack behavior when they are again placed in social situations, and meprobamate will reduce fighting here. Electric foot shock will induce fighting in pairs of rats, and meprobamate is effective in this situation as well.

In studies of this kind, meprobamate has often been compared with chlorpromazine, barbiturates, and benzodiazepines. Upon such a comparison, meprobamate is invariably found to be the least potent. There is some controversy about the specificity of the behavioral effects induced by these various drug groups. All of the drugs are sedatives, but, at least in the case of meprobamate, the anxiety-reducing effects are correlated with the ability to induce muscle relaxation.

Barbiturates also induce muscle relaxation; unlike the barbiturates, meprobamate has an anti-anxiety effect at doses that do not impair motor or intellectual performance. Chlordiazepoxide is generally thought to be unique in its selective taming effect, but there is not even agreement on this point.

Spontaneous locomotor activity is used extensively in behavioral pharmacology to assess the general depressant or stimulant properties of drugs. Such activity is thought to be a useful index when the specificity of the effect of a drug on behavior is being evaluated. Spontaneous motor activity is itself a complex of several behaviors including, for example, locomotion and exploration. The nature of the apparatus in which it is measured itself determines the nature of the spontaneous motor activity. Thus, whereas meprobamate with most measures of spontaneous motor activity produces the expected depression, experiments have been reported in which the converse was true. If mice are kept in glass beakers after injection of meprobamate, and before their activity is measured, then an increase in spontaneous motor activity is reported.

Cook and Kelleher (1963) reviewed the effect of meprobamate on a wide range of behaviors controlled by schedules of positive reinforcement and found it to have, in general, rate-increasing effects. The low rates of responding engendered by a DRL schedule are markedly reversed by meprobamate. Inter-response times are shortened, and reinforcements are thus lost. Other low rates of responding, e.g., FI 5-minute and VI 1.5-minute schedules were also increased. Rates of bar pressing for brain stimulation are also increased by meprobamate.

These rate-increasing effects of meprobamate can be obtained in monkeys, as Cook and Kelleher (1962) showed, using a multiple FI 10 and FR 30 schedule with interposed time-outs. Responding was also markedly increased by 50-199 mg/kg meprobamate without any over-all loss of discrimination. These authors observe that meprobamate and chlordiazepoxide, which was included in the study, increase behavioral output without overt signs of stimulation and, in this sense at least, can be distinguished from amphetamine, which produces similar behavioral effects on these parameters.

The rate-increasing effect, however, does not extend to behavior maintained by avoidance of or escape from aversive stimuli. Unlike amphetamine, and like chlorpromazine, meprobamate depresses avoidance behavior, but its effects are much weaker than those of chlorpromazine. In the pole climbing avoidance task, Maffi (1959) has suggested that meprobamate abolishes the anticipatory pole climbing often seen before the warning signal is sounded, although it does not have a marked effect on the avoidance response itself. Chlorpromazine, by contrast, abolishes the pole climbing response at doses that interfere with this so-called "secondary conditioning" and therefore blocks avoidance behavior to a much greater extent. Similar results are obtained with non-discriminated avoidance behavior, such as the Sidman procedure and a procedure described by

Cook and Kelleher (1962) in which squirrel monkeys worked on a concurrent avoidance, fixed-ratio schedule to avoid shock and obtain food. Shocks were programmed to occur every 30 seconds, and every response postponed the shock for 30 seconds. Simultaneously, every 100 responses produced food (FR 100). Thus, two concurrent behavioral tendencies were induced, a low rate of responding sufficient to avoid shocks and a high rate to obtain food. The resultant stable pattern of responding shows that, immediately after each food reinforcement, the animal responds at a low rate that is just high enough to avoid shocks. After responding at this low rate for a period of time, the animal abruptly shifts to a high response rate that is maintained until the next food reinforcement. Chlorpromazine depresses both behaviors, and more shocks and less food are obtained. Meprobamate depresses the high rates of the fixed ratio component, but the depression of responding results in an increased delivery of shocks only at very high doses.

Finally we come to the behavioral effects of meprobamate that are unique to the minor tranquilizers—their ability to reinstate behavior suppressed by punishment. The Estes-Skinner procedure again yields equivocal results, but on the Geller procedure with immediate punishment, the effects are clear. Meprobamate (120-135 mg/kg) increases the number of shocks a rat receives, even when intense shock levels are used (Geller and Siefter, 1960).

Barbiturates used as minor tranquilizers

We shall not dwell on this topic because barbiturates as tranquilizers have been largely supplanted by more specific drugs and also because the effects of barbiturates have been described at more length in another section (p. 179).

In brief the behavioral effects elicited by small doses of barbiturates are very similar to those of meprobamate. They do not share the powerful taming effect of chlordiazepoxide, and yet they show equally powerful releasing effect on behavior suppressed by immediate punishment. Morse and Kelleher (1964) with their multiple FR/FR punishment schedule (Fig. 4-2) have shown that pentobarbital will sustain higher rates of responding in the shock component than actual removal of the shock itself. Indeed, on the basis of this effect, which is believed to reflect the anti-anxiety effect of minor tranquilizers, it could be claimed that small doses of barbiturates are as effective as small doses of the benzodiazepines.

Benzodiazepines (chlordiazepoxide, Librium; diazepam, Valium; oxazepam, Serax)

The benzodiazepines came into use only within the last 10 years and have not been as intensively studied as meprobamate or the barbiturates. Nevertheless, there are reports of the effects of chlordiazepoxide on aggression, spontaneous motor activity, positively reinforced behavior, and immediate punishment that indicate that the benzodiazepines show the same profile of behavioral effects as meprobamate.

Furthermore, with respect to the specific behavioral effects that characterize minor tranquilizers, taming and reinstatement of punished responding, chlordiazepoxide is claimed to be more potent and selective than either meprobamate or the barbiturates.

Geller, Kulak, and Seifter (1962) first described the potent anti-punishment effect of chlordiazepoxide. Their behavioral procedure was based on the work of Estes (1944). A rat was trained to lever press for a milk reward on a VI 2-minute schedule. When the lever pressing had stabilized, a tone was introduced every 15 minutes for 3 minutes, and this signaled a change from VI to continuous reinforcement. After further stabilization, every response during the tone periods produced not only reinforcement but also a shock to the feet. In this conflict situation, the immediate punishment virtually abolished responding during the tone (Fig. 4-17A). Chlordiazepoxide in doses up to 15 mg/kg reinstated responding during the shock periods without changing the responding during the "safe" VI periods (Fig. 4-17B). This may be contrasted with earlier find-

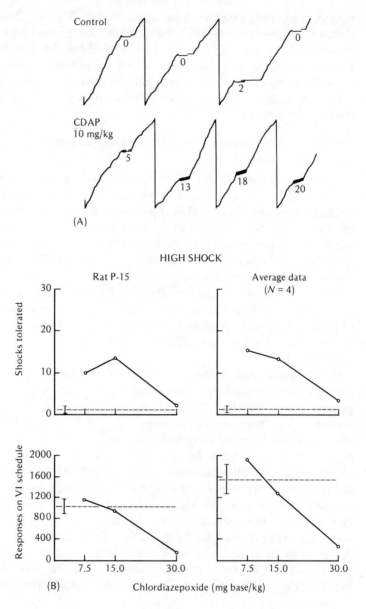

(A)

HIGH SHOCK

Rat P-15

Average data
(N = 4)

(B)

Chlordiazepoxide (mg base/kg)

ings with meprobamate and pheno- and pentobarbital. These compounds also increased punished responding, but there were invariably associated changes in the rate of non-punished VI responding.

This selectivity of the effect of chlordiazepoxide in behavioral situations involving shock was also noted by Cook and Kelleher (1962) using a concurrent avoidance fixed-ratio procedure with the squirrel monkey. The monkey was shocked every 30 seconds if it did not respond to the lever. Every response postponed the shock for 30 seconds, but at the same time every 100th response (FR 100) resulted in delivery of a food pellet. Behavior on this schedule is maintained by two conditions of reinforcement: shock avoidance (negative reinforcement) and food reward (positive reinforcement). Chlordiazepoxide had a unique effect on performance, disrupting the avoidance component and increasing the shocks taken without affecting the fixed ratio performance. By contrast, meprobamate and phenobarbital eliminated the high response rates characteristic of the fixed ratio component but only increased shocks at doses that produce signs of neurotoxicity. Rats give the same response to benzodiazepines on continuous avoidance schedules, showing a significant increase in the number of shocks taken at doses well below the tranquilizing dose.

Fig. 4-17 (A) Cumulative response records showing the effects of chlordiazepoxide (CDAP) upon a punishment discrimination maintained with a high shock. The pen offsets indicate tone periods; upward pips of the pen represent responses that were simultaneously rewarded with food and punished with shock. The numbers of such responses appears under the shock period. (B) Effects of CDAP upon a punishment discrimination maintained with a high shock. *Left:* charts show the number of shocks tolerated during tones and inter-trial VI rates for an individual rat under each drug condition. The drug points are averages for three injections. *Right:* charts show the same data averaged for four rats. Dotted lines, control values (individual data $N = 36$, grouped data $N = 144$). I---, two mean standard deviations. These means were computed by averaging the mean standard deviations of four rats, each based on thirty-six control observations. (Reproduced from Geller et al., 1962.)

TABLE 4-3

MINIMUM EFFECTIVE DOSES AND DOSE RANGE RATIO IN THE CONTINUOUS AVOIDANCE PROCEDURE

Compound	Route of admin.	Rats Shock rate increase (MED, mg/kg)	Rats Escape failure (MED, mg/kg.)	Rats Dose range ratio	Route of admin.	Squirrel monkeys Shock rate increase (MED, mg/kg)	Squirrel monkeys Escape failure (MED, mg/kg)	Squirrel monkeys Dose range ratio
Chlordiazepoxide	p.o.	5.2	60.0	—	p.o.	1.0	29.0	29.0
	i.p.	4.2	18.0	3.8				
Diazepam	p.o.	20.0	120.0	5.2	p.o.	1.0	33.0	33.0
	i.p.	10.0	67.0	5.5				
Nitrazepam	i.p.	0.81	14.0	19.0	—			
Phenobarbital	s.c.	30.0	61.0	2.1	p.o.	80.0	80.0	1.2
Methyprylon	s.c.	25.0	41.0	1.8				
Hexobarbital	s.c.	42.0	75.0	1.7				
Emylcamate	i.p.	56.0	78.0	1.2				
Pentobarbital	s.c.	12.0	18.0	1.1	p.o.	10.0	20.0	1.5
Chlormezanone	i.p.	62.0	70.0	1.1				
Meprobamate	i.p.	103.0	105.0	1.0	p.o.	200.0	200.0	—
	p.o.	250.0	300.0	1.2				
Chlorpromazine	p.o.	5.4	8.2	1.5	p.o.	2.0	2.5	1.3
	s.c.	0.21	0.62	3.4				
	i.p.	1.1	2.1	1.8				
Trifluorperazine	s.c.	0.03	0.05	1.9				

(Reproduced from Zbinden and Randall, 1967.)

Zbinden and Randall (1967) point out that chlordiazepoxide and oxazepam (0.05 mg/kg) can abolish the ability of iproniazid to accentuate the stimulatory effect of tetrabenazine on continuous avoidance behavior (Fig. 4-6b). This is an important test because, although the benzodiazepines do have pronounced effects on Sidman and discrete-trial avoidance tests, these effects are similar to the effects of the major tranquilizers. Heise and Boff (1962) proposed that the Sidman avoidance results can be used to differentiate these drug groups if a ratio measure of the minimum effective dose (MED), which causes escape failure, to the minimum dose, which just increases the number of shocks, is calculated. The benzodiazepines, with which shock increase is seen at a much lower dose than escape failure, give a high ratio, whereas for chlorpromazine these doses are very similar. This comparison also emphasizes the specificity of benzodiazepines in aversive situations because the other minor tranquilizers (meprobamate and barbiturates) closely resemble the neuroleptics when the MED ratio values are considered (Table 4-3).

There are some species differences in the responses to benzodiazepines. Cats, for example, show pronounced muscle relaxation at very low doses. Scheckel (1965) has used delayed matching of colors as an anxiety-inducing behavioral procedure with rhesus monkeys. The matching delay is increased in an orderly way each time the animal correctly matches colors at the existing delay between cue sample and choices. Very small doses of chlordiazepoxide (0.3 mg/kg) significantly increase the delay that can be tolerated (Fig. 4-18).

It is now fashionable to try to account for the apparently specific behavioral effects of certain psychoactive drugs in terms of the so-called "base-line" phenomenon discussed in Chapter 3. Chlorpromazine, for example, which is thought to interact more strongly with behavior controlled by shock than by positive reinforcement, can be shown to affect the two behavioral base lines equally if they are adjusted to control the same rate of ongoing behavior.

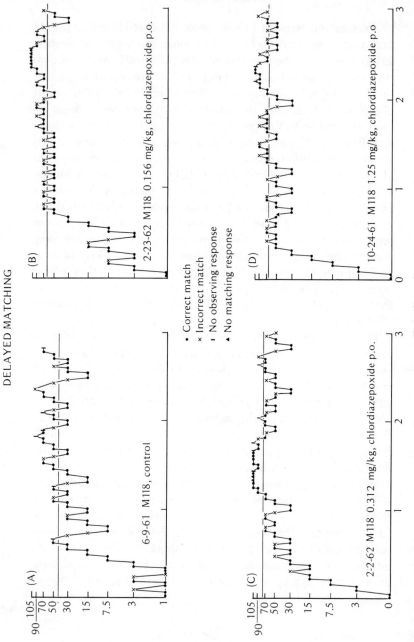

DELAYED MATCHING

- • Correct match
- × Incorrect match
- ┃ No observing response
- ▲ No matching response

(A) 6-9-61 M118, control

(B) 2-23-62 M118 0.156 mg/kg, chlordiazepoxide p.o.

(C) 2-2-62 M118 0.312 mg/kg, chlordiazepoxide p.o.

(D) 10-24-61 M118 1.25 mg/kg, chlordiazepoxide p.o

Delay interval (seconds)

Time (hours)

Wuttke and Kelleher (1970) have suggested the same baseline phenomenon occurs with the benzodiazepines. In their procedure, one group of pigeons responded under a 5-minute interval schedule of food presentation, with every 30th response producing an electric shock (punishment group). Another group responded under the same schedule of food presentation but without electric shock (non-punishment group). Both groups of birds showed the usual fixed-interval pattern of responding, although the average rate of responding was much lower in the punishment group. The lowest rates at the start of the non-punished FI, however, were comparable to the highest rates at the end of the punished FI. The benzodiazepines, chlordiazepoxide, diazepam, and nitrazepam, were compared, and all were found to markedly increase responding on the punishment schedule. But increased responding was also seen on the non-punishment schedule. These rate-increasing effects were analyzed in relation to their respective base lines, and, when this was taken into account, the authors concluded that the effects of the benzodiazepines are to increase low rates of responding, whether they are associated with punishment or reinforcement.

One is reluctant to accept the conclusion that there is not a special relationship between the benzodiazepines and punishment, and more recent results argue against the conclusions described above. First, Wuttke and Kelleher used separate groups of animals for the punishment and non-punishment schedules. McMillan (1973a), however, trained pigeons on a multiple FI

Fig. 4-18 The effect of small doses of chlordiazepoxide on a rhesus monkey in a delayed matching procedure. Each panel shows performance during a 3-hour session. Each point shows the result of a single trial. When the animal made correct responses on two consecutive trials at one delay, the delay presented on the next trial automatically increased one step. Incorrect responses or the lack of an observing response decreased the delay one step. Horizontal lines in each panel are drawn through the average limit of delay. The ordinate (duration of delay interval) is logarithmically scaled. (Reproduced from Zbinden and Randall, 1967.)

5-minute/FI 5-minute reinforcement schedule with red and green key lights. Subsequently, every response during one component of the multiple schedule produced an electric shock suppressing response rates during that part of the schedule. Chlordiazepoxide, diazepam, and oxazepam all increased the low rates of punished and unpunished responding, but the rate-increasing effect was greater for punished responses. The conclusion is that other variables can modify the rate-dependent effects of the benzodiazepines and perhaps these "other variables" relate specifically to drug interactions with punished behavior.

Miczek (1973) has approached this same problem in a rather different way. It has been suggested that a system of cholinergic neurons in the limbohypothalamic circuits may be involved in the suppression of behavior consequent upon punishment or non-reinforcement. The ventromedial nucleus of the hypothalamus is thought to be the center of this system, and cholinomimetic and anticholinergic drugs, if injected locally into this nucleus, intensify or abolish such inhibition of behavior. Interestingly, benzodiazepines injected through the same cannula have been shown to act like cholinergic antagonists and reinstate punished responding. Miczek investigated the rate-dependent hypothesis of benzodiazepine action within this framework. He used three different methods of inhibiting responding: (a) immediate punishment of operant responses; (b) non-reinforcement in the presence of an S^Δ; and (c) immediate punishment of a consummatory response. Chlordiazepoxide attenuated the suppression responses induced by immediate punishment but not those associated with non-reinforcement. The conclusion is that "it appears unlikely that the rate-dependency principles can completely account for the observed punishment attenuating effect" of the benzodiazepines.

On the basis of such evidence, one may conclude that the benzodiazepines are a unique group of anti-anxiety drugs. Their releasing effect on punished responding is not, in fact, as great as that obtained with barbiturates. Unlike barbiturates, however, which show in addition the full range of CNS depressant activity, benzodiazepines have a narrow range of behavioral effects, particularly in relation to aversive stimuli.

The benzodiazepines are also reported to exert a specific effect on a form of abnormal behavior induced by adventitious punishment that was originally described by Maier (1949). Rats were given an insoluble problem in a Lashley jumping stand and punished randomly as they performed. Fixated behavior, which took the form of position habits, i.e., jumping persistently to one side, emerged. When a soluble brightness discrimination task was subsequently presented, the rats continued to show the "fixated" position habit, although their jump latencies indicated that they in fact "knew" when they were jumping to the correct stimulus. Chlordiazepoxide further reduced the latency to the positive stimulus in a similar study (Feldman, 1964). More recently, the experiment was repeated on monkeys trained to press an illuminated key (Feldman and Freen, 1966). The spatial position of the lighted key and the reward were randomly programmed, and the animal was punished with tail shock; after 4 days of this procedure, the monkeys showed fixated responses under either stimulus or position control. They were then given a soluble problem, which was the reverse of their fixated response. As in the rat study, chlordiazepoxide lowered response latencies to the positive stimulus, although the monkeys persisted in the fixated response and were unable to learn the discrimination in more than one thousand trials.

ANTIPSYCHOTIC DRUGS

Classification and neuropharmacological properties

Introduction

The discovery of drugs that are effective in the treatment of psychotic illnesses has been perhaps the most important psychopharmacological event of the second half of the 20th century.

Behavioral Pharmacology

SELECTED PHENOTHIAZINE DERIVATIVES

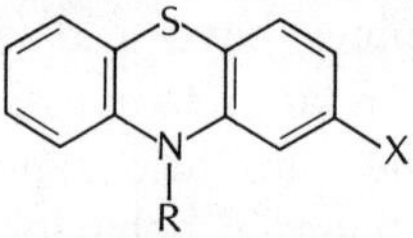

Nonproprietary name	X	R	Antipsychotic dose range* (mg/day)
Promethazine	H	$CH_2CH(CH_3)N(CH_3)_2$	—
Diethazine	H	$(CH_2)_2N(C_2H_5)_2$	—
Promazine	H	$(CH_2)_3N(CH_3)_2$	200-1000
Chlorpromazine	Cl	$(CH_2)_3N(CH_3)_2$	400-1600
Thioridazine	SCH_3	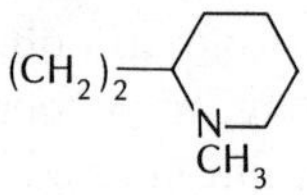 $(CH_2)_2$ ⟨piperidine N-CH_3⟩	400-1600
Triflupromazine	CF_3	$(CH_2)_3N(CH_3)_2$	75-300
Prochlorperazine	Cl	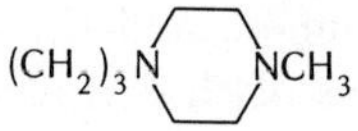 $(CH_2)_3N$ ⟨piperazine⟩ NCH_3	30-200
Trifluoperazine	CF_3	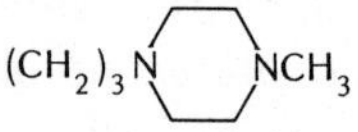 $(CH_2)_3N$ ⟨piperazine⟩ NCH_3	6-30
Perphenazine	Cl	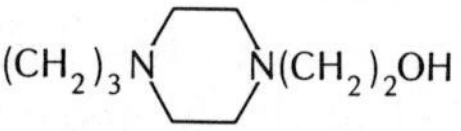 $(CH_2)_3N$ ⟨piperazine⟩ $N(CH_2)_2OH$	12-64
Fluphenazine	CF_3	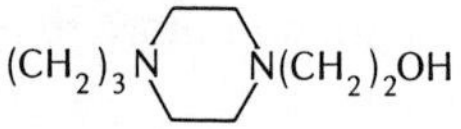 $(CH_2)_3N$ ⟨piperazine⟩ $N(CH_2)_2OH$	2-20

*For adult hospitalized or severely disturbed patients

Fig. 4-19   The phenothiazine neuroleptic drugs.

The dramatic impact that such drugs have had on the treatment of hitherto intractable psychotic illnesses has been responsible in large part for the rapid development of psychopharmacology as an academic discipline in the last 20 years. Before the advent of the antipsychotics, usually known as NEUROLEPTICS, virtually no successful forms of physical treatment of schizophrenia were known, and many mental hospitals had been largely custodial in function. Since the introduction and widespread use of neuroleptic drugs, the in-patient population of such hospitals has declined dramatically. This phenomenon has become so common that in the United Kingdom such custodial hospitals will gradually be phased out in coming years.

What are the neuroleptics?

The first widely used drug for the treatment of psychoses was the phenothiazine, CHLORPROMAZINE (Fig. 4-19), and it remains the most important drug in clinical use today. It is estimated that more than 50 million patients around the world have received treatment with this drug in the 25 years since its introduction into clinical practice. The striking successes obtained with chlorpromazine led to investigations of several hundreds of related phenothiazines and other chemical congeners, many of which have proved useful in clinical practice (Fig. 4-19). Not only phenothiazines, but the related thioxanthenes (e.g., FLUPENTHIXOL) and the chemically unrelated butyrophenones (e.g., HALOPERIDOL) have proved to be neuroleptic (Fig. 4-20). This is not to say that all phenothiazines and all butyrophenones are neuroleptic; this is far from the case, since quite small structural changes in these compounds can cause a complete loss of neuroleptic activity. For example, all the active members of the phenothiazine series have a chlorine, fluorine, or thio-substituent in the 3-position of the phenothiazine ring; such substituents in any other position on the aromatic ring, for example, the adjacent 2-position, are quite ineffective, although these analogues have very similar physical and chemical properties. It is clear, therefore, that the neuroleptic activity of the active compounds in these series is a highly specific molecular property and is not simply related to lipid solubility or other physicochemical properties of the compounds, as is the case for local and general anesthetics, for example.

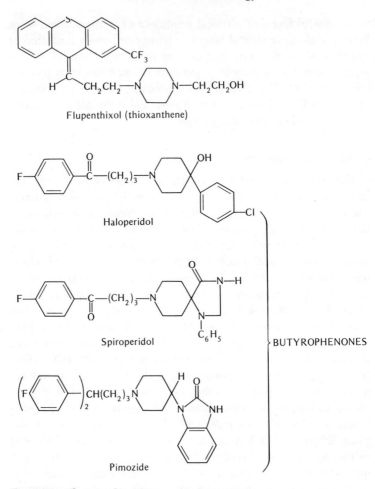

Fig. 4-20   The non-phenothizine neuroleptic drugs.

The neuroleptics are usually administered orally, are well absorbed, and penetrate readily into the CNS. Recently a new method of administering such drugs has been developed; this involves the intramuscular injection of water-insoluble lipid ester derivatives of the drug in an oil base. Such an injection acts as a "depot" from which the parent drug is gradually released into the bloodstream, thus sustaining therapeutic levels of the active drug in the body for periods as long as a month after injection. By using such depot injections, out-patient treatment of schizophrenia has become a practical and rapidly growing possibility.

Are the neuroleptics really antipsychotic?

There is a great deal of confusion about the specificity of action of phenothiazines and other neuroleptics in the treatment of schizophrenia and other psychoses. It has been popularly assumed that the drugs do not really alleviate the symptoms of the psychotic illness, but merely sedate or "tranquilize" otherwise recalcitrant patients. Current evidence, however, argues overwhelmingly against this view and suggests that the drugs do have a very specific antipsychotic action not found in other classes of sedative drugs, such as the barbiturates or the antianxiety agents (see Snyder, 1974). On a large scale, carefully controlled multi-hospital series of collaborative studies, sponsored by the Veterans Administration (VA) and the National Institutes of Mental Health (NIMH) in the United States, the effects of phenothiazines and barbiturates were compared in several thousand patients (Klein and Davis, 1969). Phenothiazines were more effective in the treatment of schizophrenia than the placebo in a large majority of the studies, whereas phenobarbital was no better than the placebo in any of the studies. Extensive trials of such anti-anxiety drugs as chlordiazepoxide and diazepam have also shown these agents to be ineffective in the treatment of schizophrenia. The VA-NIMH studies also showed that the phenothiazines were most effective in treating those features of schizophrenia that have been classified by Bleuler (1911) as the "fundamental" features of the disease, whereas other symptoms classified as "accessory" or unrelated specifically to the disease responded somewhat less consistently to phenothiazines and symptoms unrelated to schizophrenia per se did not respond at all (Table 4-4). There is thus a large

TABLE 4-4
DIFFERENTIAL RESPONSE OF SCHIZOPHRENIC SYMPTOMS
TO PHENOTHIAZINES

Bleuler's classification	Response
Fundamental Symptoms	
Thought disorder	+++
Blunted affect	+++
Withdrawal	+++
Autistic behavior	+++
Accessory Symptoms	
Hallucinations	++
Paranoid ideation	+
Grandiosity	+
Hostility–Belligerence	0
Nonschizophrenic Symptoms	
Anxiety–Tension–Agitation	0
Guilt–Depression	0

(Adapted from Klein and Davis, 1969.)

body of evidence to suggest that the neuroleptics exert a unique pharmacological action in schizophrenic patients. This does not necessarily mean that these drugs act directly on whatever hypothetical biochemical defect may be primarily responsible for the psychotic state, but it does mean that a better understanding of the site of action of the neuroleptics could prove very valuable in understanding the neural mechanisms underlying this psychosis. Nor is it true that neuroleptics "cure" schizophrenia; there is a high incidence of remission in patients successfully treated with these drugs who then stop taking them. Nevertheless, many schizophrenic patients can be maintained in a state of sufficient normality to sustain a normal life out of the hospital by continuous treatment with neuroleptics.

Neuropharmacological actions of neuroleptics in animals

Chlorpromazine has been the subject of a very large number of pharmacological studies, and it has a rather wide range of phar-

macological activities. It is a moderately potent antagonist of
α-adrenoceptors in peripheral tissue, although not of β-adrenoceptors. It also has weak anticholinergic, antihistaminic, and
anti-5-HT activity. In addition, chlorpromazine and various related phenothiazines are quite potent local anesthetics, a property undoubtedly related to the high lipid solubility of these
compounds, which results in their being concentrated by the
lipid-rich membranes of nerves and other cells. These properties, however, are not shared by all neuroleptics, and it is only
recently that a unifying hypothesis for the mode of action of
such drugs has been formulated. Regardless of whatever secondary and varied pharmacological properties individual drugs
in this group may have, they share one common and probably
crucial neuropharmacological property, namely, that they are
all antagonists of the action of DA at CNS receptor sites (see
Snyder, 1974 for references). The evidence for this stems from
a variety of experiments. First, biochemical studies have shown
that all neuroleptics accelerate the rate of release and turnover of DA in the animal brain. This is revealed by an increased
concentration of the DA metabolite, homovanillic acid, an increased rate of conversion of labeled tyrosine to DA, and an
accelerated rate of disappearance of labeled DA synthesized
from tyrosine in the brain following the administration of neuroleptic drugs. The increased turnover of DA is thought to be a
consequence of a blockade of DA receptors induced by the
neuroleptic drugs, leading to a reflex increase in the rate of firing of dopaminergic neurons, with a consequent increase in their
metabolic utilization of DA. The increased turnover of DA does
not occur in the rat striatum, for example, if the dopaminergic
axon pathway from the substantia nigra is sectioned just before
the neuroleptic drug is given.

More direct evidence for a blockade of DA receptors by
neuroleptics has been obtained by neurophysiological studies.
In these studies, it has been possible to show that, when such
neuroleptics as chlorpromazine or haloperidol are applied via
micro-electrodes, they antagonize the inhibitory effects of DA

on neurons in the basal ganglia if DA is iontophoretically applied from another barrel of the same electrode. These experiments have proved technically difficult to perform because the local anesthetic properties of the neuroleptic drugs tend to depress neuronal activity in a non-specific manner. By using very small doses of the applied drug, however, specific anti-DA properties of neuroleptics have been detected (York, 1974). Other neurophysiological studies have shown, by directly recording from the DA neurons in the substantia nigra, that neuroleptics do indeed lead to a sustained increase in the rate of firing of these cells, as suggested by the biochemical experiments (Bunney and Aghajanian, 1974).

As discussed below, the anti-dopaminergic properties of the neuroleptic drugs are also demonstrated in behavioral experiments in which these substances have been found to potently antagonize the effects of such drugs as APOMORPHINE and amphetamine, which are thought to exert their actions by stimulating DA receptors.

Biochemical studies have recently opened a second line of approach to studies of CNS DA receptors by the discovery that DA stimulates the synthesis of cyclic AMP when it is added to homogenates of basal ganglia or retina; this effect is not seen with homogenates of other brain regions that do not contain dopaminergic nerve terminals. The DA-sensitive adenylate cyclase activity of basal ganglia or retina seems a useful model for studies of drugs that stimulate (apomorphine) or antagonize (neuroleptics) CNS DA receptors. The neuroleptics are potent inhibitors of this adenylate cyclase, whereas related phenothiazines or other drugs that lack neuroleptic properties are inactive. It seems likely that DA exerts its action in the brain by stimulating cyclic AMP production in receptive postsynaptic cells, and this may be the primary step antagonized by the neuroleptic drugs.

Many neuroleptics, of course, have other important neuropharmacological properties. Many are NE antagonists at α-adrenoceptors, which probably explains why, in addition to causing increases in the turnover of brain dopamine, they have similar effects in stimulating the turnover of brain NE. Chlorpromazine is relatively unspecific in its action on DA metabolism; it is almost as active in its effect on NE turnover in the brain. Some neuroleptic drugs, however, including haloperidol, fluphenazine, flupenthixol, and pimozide, seem to be much more specific in their DA antagonist effects, since they have little effect on NE turnover in the CNS. The secondary neuropharmacological properties of the neuroleptics may be of great importance, since these properties may explain some of the undesirable side effects of long-term treatment with these drugs. Many, and perhaps all, neuroleptics lead to a snydrome of extrapyramidal motor disorders similar to that seen in Parkinson's disease, characterized by muscular rigidity, tremor, and akinesia (the absence or paucity of power of voluntary movement). This undesirable side effect, however, seems to be produced more readily by some neuroleptic drugs than by others; perhaps it is not simply related to the anti-DA properties of the drugs, but to a combination of their anti-DA, anti-NE, and anticholinergic properties. Parkinson's disease is commonly treated with anticholinergic drugs. It has been suggested that the neuroleptics that are least likely to cause the extrapyramidal side effect are the ones that combine anti-dopaminergic and anticholinergic properties, since the latter would tend to counteract the Parkinson-like symptoms.

Behavioral actions of the neuroleptics

In the absence of any appropriate animal model of schizophrenia, the task in behavioral pharmacology is to discover some behavioral parameters with which to characterize and differentiate the highly specific antipsychotic drugs from other psychoactive agents. The phenothiazines and related drugs are depressants, but it is clear, at least from the clinical data, that their antipsychotic potency is not related to their depressant action. Large doses of barbiturates, despite their potent depressant action, have been found to be quite ineffective in relieving the fundamental symptoms of schizophrenia.

Phenothiazines

Chlorpromazine is the best studied example of this class of neuroleptic drugs, and it has the general effect of abolishing "behavioral tone" in almost any situation. For example, it reduces spontaneous locomotor activity. This is the case in whatever apparatus the spontaneous locomotor activity is measured, provided sufficiently large doses of the drug are used. It may be that more attention should be paid to the manner in which motor activity is measured. It is possible, for example, that wheel-running is controlled to a greater extent by proprioceptive feedback than free cage activity and could thus be expected to show a different profile of drug sensitivity. Indeed, stimulation of wheel running in rats after chlorpromazine administration has been reported. Phenothiazines antagonize amphetamine-induced stimulation of locomotor behavior presumably, as we have seen, because they block NE and DA receptors. The basal ganglia are thought to be involved in this antagonism because the appearance of extrapyramidal motor symptoms reminiscent of Parkinson's disease is one of the side effects associated with chronic phenothiazine treatment. The antipsychotic effect appears to be correlated with this akinesia and rigidity, and handwriting tests are often used to titrate the dosage on this basis. It seems that, in order to achieve the maximum antipsychotic effect, a degree of undesirable extrapyramidal side effects must be tolerated. The search continues for effective antipsychotics that do not have such side effects.

An effect of chlorpromazine on conditioned behavior was described in an early account of its pharmacology by Courvoisier et al. (1953). A pole-climbing test for the rat was used. The animal was placed on floor bars of a cage and a tone sounded for 10 seconds before the floor was electrified. An insulated pole from floor to ceiling provided a means of escape from or avoidance of the foot shock. After a few trials, the rat climbed the pole when the tone sounded in anticipation of the shock, an example of avoidance learning. After moderate doses of chloropromazine, the rat no longer responded to the tone but did respond to the shock by climbing the pole. Thus, avoidance was abolished, but escape behavior remained. Dews and Morse (1961) interpret the loss of avoidance as an inability to make a discriminated conditioned response to two stimuli. Avoidance is more readily suppressed than escape; in the pole-climbing situation four times the dose for avoidance suppression was required to suppress escape. This differential effect is seen in similar situations. Two-chamber shuttle boxes provide another method for dissociating avoidance and escape. The rat is placed in one chamber, a conditioned stimulus is presented and followed by a foot shock. This can be avoided if the animal moves to the other chamber during the conditioned stimulus or escaped from if movement to the other chamber does not occur until the shock is presented. Verhave et al. (1959) describe a test in which wheel-turning provided the avoidance and escape responses and reports that 4 mg/kg chlorpromazine causes an 80% loss of avoidance and only a 5% loss of escape in the rat. This differential effect of chlorpromazine and other antipsychotics may be compared with the effects of barbiturates that depress avoidance and escape equally.

Several experimental results have suggested that chlorpromazine reduces the ability of exteroceptive or interoceptive stimuli to signal that responses are relevant or irrelevant. If pigeons are trained in the presence of a red light to peck for food on an FR 50 schedule and, when the key color changes to blue, the first peck after 15 minutes is rewarded (FI 15 minutes), the control performance shows high rates of FR responding followed by the scalloped pattern typical of FI schedules. After 3 mg/kg of chlorpromazine, the difference in the pattern of responding to the two stimuli is reduced. High bursts of responding occurred early in fixed intervals, for example. The pattern of responding under the influence of the drug was very similar to that observed when the discriminative stimuli were switched off during control sessions.

The apparent loss of behavioral response with phenothiazines, therefore, seems to be due to a loss of response to certain controlling stimuli in the environment. Presumably, the dampening effect on stimulus control will depend on how important the stimulus is for controlling behavior, a weak discriminative stimulus being abolished more easily than a strong one. Some of the experiments of Maffii (1959) using the pole-climbing technique demonstrate this. It was observed that well-trained rats climb the pole even before the conditioned stimulus is presented, and that there are thus three discriminative stimuli in the test: (a) general environment of the box, (b) warning signal, and (c) shock. The effective doses of chlorpromazine for eliminating responses to these three stimuli are 1.75, 11.6, and 30.0 mg/kg. The shock is the strongest S^D and the most difficult to disrupt.

Dews and Morse (1961) have suggested that antipsychotics "manipulate the relationship between the environment and the animal," and this hypothesis encompasses the results obtained with such drugs on food reinforcement, shock-avoidance, and shock-escape, although it undermines the widely held view that there is something fundamental about the differential effect of chlorpromazine on avoidance and escape behavior. Courvoisier et al. (1953) thought, for example, that unconditioned responses remained after chlorpromazine, while conditioned responses were lost; but, in fact, an escape response is a conditioned response just as an avoidance response is, insofar as it may not occur with the first few presentations of the shock.

Chlorpromazine will also reduce behavior maintained by positive reinforcement, as opposed to suppression of responses to aversive stimuli. Food and water intake, sexual behavior, and lever pressing for electric stimulation of the limbo hypothalamic system or for self-administration of such reinforcing drugs as cocaine and amphetamine by the monkey are all reduced by chlorpromazine. It has often been suggested that antipsychotics have a greater effect on behavior maintained by aversive reinforcers than by positive reinforcers, but this does not actually seem to be the case. Wenzel (1964) made this proposal after comparing the effect of reserpine on food-reinforced and shock-avoidance behavior in the cat. It was claimed that the drug increased response latencies for shock avoidance more than responses for food, but, in fact, the pre-drug latencies for shock were already double those for food. The more parsimonious interpretation is that if response probability is matched chlorpromazine affects shock avoidance and shock-escape. Morse and Kelleher (1964) maintained squirrel monkeys on FI/FR shock-escape and FI/FR food-reinforcement. The behavioral base lines were indistinguishable and so were the dose-dependent decreases in both behaviors after chlorpromazine. Motivation variables, therefore, seem irrelevant in the characterization of antipsychotic drugs.

Most of the clinically described effects of chlorpromazine—loss of initiative and reactivity, reduction of tension and compulsiveness—can be translated into terms of stimulus control manipulation. One might suppose that social behavior, which is precisely determined by a sequence of external stimuli, would be a sensitive index of antipsychotic activity. Silverman (1965) has used such an index in the rat, for which more than forty elements of social behavior can be distinguished and measured. There was no evidence that chlorpromazine reduced all behavior by causing a general motor depression. Nor was there evidence of a general loss of responsiveness to the environment: exploration was unchanged. But the response tendencies induced by certain exteroceptive cues associated with other rats were markedly changed. Mating and aggression were reduced and escape behavior increased. If rats or mice are socially stimulated in crowded living quarters, they are killed more readily by amphetamine. Chlorpromazine antagonizes this effect and the stronger the social stimulation the greater the antagonism. The LD_{50} of amphetamine in isolated mice is increased from 111 to 144 mg/kg, but, in mice housed in groups of three, the LD_{50} for amphetamine rises from 15 to 121 mg/kg after chlorpromazine. Chlorpromazine appears to reduce the responsiveness of individual mice to the stimuli engendered by other mice. There may be a straightforward pharmacological explanation of this interesting effect. Sensory stimuli and amphetamine induce arousal, release of endogenous amines, and increased activity in amine-sensitive neuronal systems. The greater the induced activity, the greater effect the amine-blocking actions of chlorpromazine will have in restoring amine homeostasis in such synaptic mechanisms.

Although the sedative effects of the phenothiazines are their most dramatic behavioral effect, it is doubtful if their antipsychotic action depends on sedation (see p. 241). For this reason, species (like the pigeon) in which behavior is stimulated by these drugs are useful in studies of their more subtle behavioral effects. For example, their apparent failure to reinstate punished responding in the rat was questioned by Morse and Kelleher (1964) on the assumption that their sedative effect might mask suppression attentuation. They, therefore, tested pigeons on their FR 30/FR 30 punishment multiple schedule and found that, although 30 mg/kg of chlorpromazine increased FR 30 responding, there was still no reinstatement of behavior suppressed in the alternate punishment segments (Fig. 4-21). The pigeon has also proved a useful model for studying the effect of phenothiazines on exteroceptive discriminative control. For example, Cook and Kelleher (1962) found that phenothiazines *increase* responses to a stimulus key that provides information about the availability of reinforcement. Pigeons were trained to peck each of two keys, one food-producing, one stimulus-producing. Positive and negative periods alternated. During

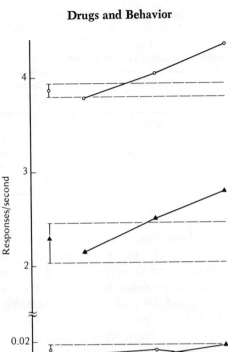

Fig. 4-21 Effects of chlorpromazine on rates of responding under the 30-response, fixed-ratio procedure in which nonpunishment and punishment components alternate. The points at the left of each record are means of control determinations; the solid vertical lines and dashed horizontal lines indicates the ranges of control observations. The ordinate has been broken to expand the scale at the lower values. The two curves above the break show the rates of responding for two pigeons in the nonpunishment component. Circles, pigeon 234, which had a control rate of 3.9 responses/ second; triangles, pigeon 235, which had a control rate of only 2.3 responses/second. The two curves below the break show rates of responding on the punishment components for the same birds. Note that chlorpromazine produced graded increases in rates of responding in nonpunishment components but had no effect on responding in punishment components. (Reproduced from Kelleher and Morse, 1964.)

TABLE 4-5

RESULTS WITH PHENOTHIAZINE-RELATED COMPOUNDS

	Increases stimulus key responding	Decreases food-producing responses
Chlorpromazine	Yes	Yes
Prochlorperazine	Yes	Yes
Trifluoperazine	No—decreases	Yes
Promazine	Yes	No effect
Triflupromazine	Yes	Yes

these times, both keys were white but pecking the food key during the positive periods produced reinforcement on a 100 VR schedule; during the negative period no reinforcement was produced. Pecking of the stimulus key was programmed so that, during the food period, 20 pecks changed both keys to green and, during the negative period, to red. This behavior to the stimulus key produced information about the availability of food. Under normal conditions, responses are distributed between the two keys. Chlorpromazine increases stimulus key responding and decreases responding for food, so that the discrimination between positive and negative periods was sharpened. Similar results were produced by related phenothiazines, which were being investigated by Smith, Kline & French at that time (see Table 4-5).

It seems that the ability of the phenothiazines to modulate the control of external stimuli over behavior may be a better index of their therapeutic value in treating psychotic behavior than their sedative effects, although we do not have information on the effects of recently developed, specific DA-blocking antipsychotics on this test. Emley and Hutchinson (1972) have studied the effects of chlorpromazine on squirrel monkeys exposed to an adventitious shock procedure for inducing aggression (see p. 41). Shocks to the tail every 4 minutes induce aggression, which manifests itself as hose biting during the shock and somatomotor activity in anticipation of the shock, which results in lever pressing. Chlorpromazine decreases hose biting under these conditions but also increases the anticipatory motor behavior and lever pressing. Major tranquilizers are used in humans to relieve the disruptive emotional excesses induced by irritating environmental events. They could act by depressing such behavior, and the attenuation of hose biting suggests that they do. In addition, they could also enhance attentional or anticipatory behaviors necessary for reward and thereby reduce frustration. These results suggest that they do both, shifting an organism's response tendency from post-event irritability and aggression toward pre-event anticipation, a prerequisite for the acquisition and maintenance of rewarded performance.

Butyrophenones

These antipsychotic drugs were introduced in the mid 1960's and have not been investigated as extensively as the phenothiazines. As far as the studies have progressed, however, the behavioral properties of these drugs appear very similar to those of the phenothiazines. The butyrophenones are generally more specific and more active as DA antagonists than chlorpromazine, and this may explain their potency in blocking such drug effects as amphetamine-induced stereotypy, which are thought to involve DA receptors primarily. Hanson et al. (1966) have compared the relative potency of a series of depressant drugs on Sidman avoidance in the squirrel monkey. Haloperidol was found to be 6.74 times as potent as chlorpromazine. It is interesting that the butyrophenones stimulate spontaneous motor behavior at very low doses, whereas the action of the phenothiazines is purely depressant. It is possible that dissociation of these two groups of antipsychotics will not be possible behaviorally, but it may be more readily accomplished in terms of their amine antagonistic actions.

HALLUCINOGENIC DRUGS AND CANNABIS

Classification and neuropharmacological properties

This is a remarkably diverse collection of drugs, and it is not easy to define the term "hallucinogenic." Perhaps the term "phantasticant" would give a more encompassing description of these agents, which share a common action in man in leading to a change in consciousness involving a change in reality, often associated with hallucinations. As Ray (1972) puts it, "The phantasticants . . . replace the present world with an alternative world—one that is equally real but different. Both the drug-induced and the nondrug world can be attended to at the same time, and there is memory for the drug-induced reality after the drug effect diminishes." We have chosen to include marijuana and the tetrahydrocannabinols in this section, although these drugs do not fit clearly into the group.

Considering the popular attention the hallucinogens have received in recent years, and the considerable social impact their widespread use has had, we remain remarkably ignorant of the scientific basis for the action of any of these drugs (Hoffer and Osmond, 1967).

d-Lysergic acid diethylamide (LSD) and indolamine hallucinogens

The striking hallucinogenic properties of LSD have been known since 1938 when the Swiss chemist Hoffman synthesized this substance from naturally occurring lysergic acid, an alkaloid extracted from the ergot fungus that affects rye and other grains. In man, the d-isomer of LSD remains the most potent hallucinogenic substance known—100 to 500 μg alter sensory perception and the sense of reality greatly, with prominent visual hallucinations. The mode of action of LSD is still unknown, but it is likely that it acts on a 5-HT (or related indolamine) transmitter system in the brain. The LSD molecule contains an indole nucleus, as does 5-HT (see Fig. 2-18). Gadum and his colleagues found that LSD was a potent antagonist of the action of 5-HT on intestinal smooth muscle, and it was originally thought that the CNS activity of LSD might be related to an antagonist effect on 5-HT receptors in the CNS. This hypothesis, however, is no longer tenable. The major argument against such a proposal stems from the finding that a related substance, the bromo-derivative (Fig. 2-18) of LSD, is effective as a 5-HT antagonist in a peripheral test system but is not hallucinogenic. Bromo-LSD penetrates the blood-brain barrier, so its lack of CNS action cannot be attributed to non-penetration into the brain. Recent neurophysiological studies have shown that LSD may actually mimic the effects of 5-HT at certain synapses in the brain. Aghajanian et al. (1970) found that LSD, like 5-HT, stimulates the firing of certain brain stem neurons that receive an input from the 5-HT-containing cells in the raphe nuclei. On the other hand, also like 5-HT, LSD inhibits the rate of firing of the raphe 5-HT neurons themselves. These effects could be elicited by the administration of very small doses of LSD (10 μg/kg) systemically, or by direct iontophoretic application of exceedingly small amounts of LSD onto the neurons in the brain stem. Biochemical evidence also supports the view that LSD acts as an agonist, since it slows the rate of turnover of 5-HT in rat brain, a change consistent with the "receptor feedback" concept described in Chapter 2, by which agonist drugs are expected to slow turnover and antagonists to accelerate turnover of the CNS transmitters with whose receptors they interact. It is possible, however, that LSD affects not 5-HT neurons but some more specialized category of indolamine neurons in which the transmitter is not actually 5-HT but a related indolamine, as yet unidentified. The existence of such neurons in the raphe nuclei has been suggested by histochemical findings (Bjorklund et al., 1970).

Apart from LSD, there are a number of other indolamine

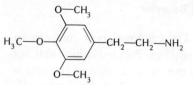

Mescaline

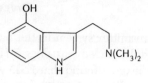

Psilocyin

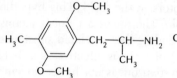

DOM (STP)
(2-amino-1-[2′,5′-dimethoxy-4′-methyl]-
phenylpropane)

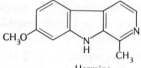

Harmine

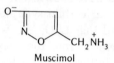

Muscimol

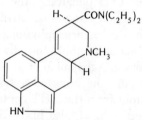

d-Lysergic acid
diethylamide (LSD)

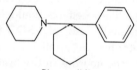

Phencyclidin
(Sernyl)

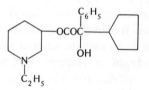

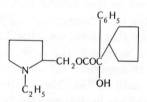

Piperidyl glycolate esters
(Ditran is a mixture of these
two compounds)

Fig. 4-22   Hallucinogenic drugs.

hallucinogens, including N-dimethyltryptamine (about 250 times less potent than LSD in man) and psilocyin. The latter is derived as the active material from psilocybin, the phosphorylated precursor present in the sacred mushrooms of Central America, which are about one-hundred times less potent than LSD. Another alkaloid, harmine, and related substances also have hallucinogenic properties (Fig. 4-22).

Tolerance to LSD develops rapidly in man, and repeated daily doses become completely ineffective after 3 to 4 days. A phenomenon known as cross-tolerance develops between LSD, psilocyin, and mescaline—meaning that after tolerance has developed to one of these drugs the others are also tolerated. The existence of cross-tolerance between several different hallucinogenic drugs is strong pharmacological evidence that they share some common mechanism of action.

Mescaline and other methoxylated phenylethylamines

The hallucinogenic properties of mescaline are well known, although the compound is, in fact, one of the least potent of the hallucinogens, requiring a dose of some 350 mg in man—or more than one thousand times the amount for LSD.

Mescaline was derived initially from the dried cactus or "peyote" used by the Aztecs and later by North American Indians in religious rites. Mescaline and many other related hallucinogenic derivatives of phenylethylamine have since been synthesized. Some of these compounds are listed in Table 4-6. The substances DDET and DOM are particularly interesting. These compounds are far more potent than mescaline, and although they seem to produce the "insight" or increased self-awareness characteristic of the LSD syndrome, they are far less effective than other hallucinogenic drugs in causing visual hallucinations. Mescaline and other hallucinogenic phenylethylamine derivatives bear an obvious structural resemblance to the catecholamine transmitters, but there is no pharmacological evidence that their CNS actions are related to an effect on adrenergic mechanisms. Since cross-tolerance develops between mescaline and

TABLE 4-6

MESCALINE AND RELATED METHOXYLATED PHENYLETHYLAMINES

Compound	Hallucinogenic potency in man[*]
Mescaline (3,4,5-trimethoxyphenylethylamine)	1
3,4,5-TMA (trimethoxyamphetamine)	2.2
2,4,6-TMA	13
2,4,5-TMA	17
2,3,6-TMA	10
2,3,5-TMA	4
2,5-DMA (dimethoxyamphetamine)	8
2,4-DMA	5
DOM (2,5-dimethoxy-4-methyl amphetamine)	50-100
DOET (2,5-dimethoxy-4-ethyl amphetamine)	100
2,4-5-MMDA (2-methoxy, 4-5-methylene dioxyamphetamine)	12
2,3-4-MMDA	10
2,3-4-MMDA	3

(Data from Snyder et al., 1970.)

[*] Potency is defined in mescaline units to indicate how many times more potent than mescaline the above compounds are in man; the average hallucinogenic dose of mescaline is 350 mg.

LSD, a common mode of action, perhaps on the indolamine systems, seems more likely.

Other hallucinogens

Many substances that are unrelated to the indolamines or the phenylethylamines have been found to be hallucinogenic. These include the compounds ibotenic acid and muscimol, isolated from the North European "magic mushroom" *Amanita muscaria* (Fig. 4-22). The pharmacological action of these compounds is obscure. Muscimol is not dissimilar to GABA structurally and has been found to inhibit CNS neurons consistent with its agonistic properties at GABA receptors. Among a series of piperidyl glycolate esters, "Ditran" (Fig. 4-20), which is a mixture of two such compounds, was found to be hallucinogenic—although this property does not appear to relate to the anticholinergic actions of the drug, since other CNS anticholinergics are not hallucinogenic. Phencyclidine, an anesthetic, also produces disorganization of thought and loss of contact with reality. The diversity of chemical structures seen in the hallucinogens does not make the pharmacologist's task easier, in trying to understand what mode of action, if any, these drugs share.

Marijuana and the synthetic tetrahydrocannabinols

The dried leaves and flowers of the hemp plant, *Cannabis sativa*, are known as marijuana. The more potent hashish is a resin derived from *Cannabis* flowers, which contain a high concentration of the psychoactive ingredients. These ingredients

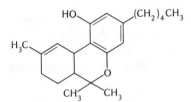

Δ^9-Trans-tetrahydrocannabinol

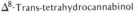

Δ^8-Trans-tetrahydrocannabinol

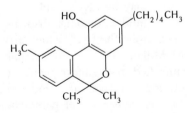

Cannabinol

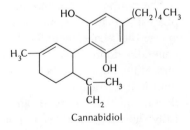

Cannabidiol

Fig. 4-23   *Cannabis sativa* derivatives.

have been chemically identified, and the principal active material is Δ9-tetrahydrocannabinol (Fig. 4-23). Very little is known of the mode of action of this and related *Cannabis* derivatives on the CNS. Δ9-Tetrahydrocannabinol apparently is metabolized and excreted only slowly in man, with as much as one-half of an injected dose of the radioactively labeled drug remaining in the body 2 days after administration. There is also some evidence that chronic drug use may induce liver hydroxylating enzymes that can convert tetrahydrocannabinol to a psychopharmacologically active hydroxylated derivative.

Behavioral pharmacology

Animal behavior studies of the hallucinogens are exceptionally difficult to interpret because of the intensely subjective nature of the effects of these substances. Although animals may indeed be subject to the visual and auditory hallucinations and bizarre perceptual changes caused by such drugs in man, this is clearly not objectively measurable. The best we can do is to attempt to determine whether such drugs induce a characteristic pattern of changes in behavior that can be observed and measured —although this must always be a poor shadow of the information that can be derived from studies in man.

Mescaline and related drugs

The symptoms of acute intoxication may be divided into two phases: the first is characterized by mild autonomic disturbances; the second includes the effects upon the CNS, which are generally depressive in nature. McMillan (1973a) reports that mescaline depresses behavior controlled by reinforcement or punishment. In the second phase, dogs and cats are rendered docile and tame. Rats are described as catatonic, yet paradoxically show hyperactivity to noises. Much higher doses appear to dampen the responses to painful stimuli. In mice, compulsive scratching has been observed, and this is antagonized by chlorpromazine.

The changed response to stimuli may also underline the aberrant conditioned avoidance behavior observed in several species after mescaline administration. Rats were trained to an avoidance response to an auditory signal to avoid electric shock. After 100 mg/kg of mescaline, they reacted to the auditory signal as if it were an electric shock, squealing and jumping. Dogs showed similar behavior to tones signaling shock to the paw.

Smythies et al. (1967) report a biphasic change in conditioned avoidance response (CAR) latencies after mescaline. Initially, 25 mg/kg causes loss of CAR with increased response latencies, but this is followed by a decrease in reaction time below control values. Substitution of either the 4- or 5-methoxy group in mescaline with an OH group abolishes the biphasic effect on CAR and produces a drug with little psychotomimetic activity in either animals or man. By contrast, modification of the molecule by introduction of a methyl group in the alpha position of the side chain yields compounds structurally related to amphetamine with potent psychotomimetic effects in both animals and man.

DOM (2,5-dimethoxy-4-methylamphetamine) is a drug that produces intense excitement and elation. Small doses produce what may well be hallucinatory behavior in cats: staring gaze, sudden jumping in the cage, and attempts to catch imaginary objects. The EEG activity after these doses is very similar to that produced by such sympathomimetic amines as amphetamine. With higher doses, motor convulsions, which cannot be antagonized by chlorpromazine, occur.

Lysergic Acid, LSD

As in the case of mescaline, the symptoms of LSD intoxication can be divided into two categories, one relating to the autonomic nervous system and the other, mood change, to the

CNS. The latter can vary from euphoria to anxiety and depression, which one perhaps depending on the individual's personailty.

The principal subjective symptoms are perceptual, and images of extraordinary complexity and plasticity are seen. On this account, the drug is termed hallucinogenic, even though the appearance of real hallucinations, i.e., formed images independent of external stimuli, are not common at usual doses. Auditory as well as visual effects are common, and intellectual processes are impaired. In subhuman primates, LSD produces hallucinatory behavior. In baboons, 10-40 μg/kg produced hyperexcitability; there was mild ataxia and grasping of non-existent objects in the air. At slightly higher doses, spatial orientation (climbing, swinging, and jumping) was impaired, but these doses did not inactivate the animals.

Parallels of the sensory and intellectual effects of LSD in man have been sought in a range of animals. Although, as Groh and Lemieux (1968) so rightly say, "there is a considerable distance on the evolutionary scale between spiders and man," it is tempting to draw parallels between their observation that LSD disrupts the highly patterned and regular web spinning of the *Aranea diademata* spider and reports of altered perception in higher animals. The sensory disturbances have prompted neurophysiological studies of the effects of the drug on the afferent sensory pathways. In the cat (Evarts, 1957), spontaneous activity in the lateral geniculate body was severely depressed by 30 μg/kg of LSD injected intra-arterially; this observation has been verified by other workers. Recently, Horn and McKay (1973) have asked more specific questions about how LSD changes the sensory receptive fields of lateral geniculate nucleus neurons. At this level in the visual system, neurons show characteristic concentric circular receptive fields in which the center either gives an "on" or "off" response to a spot light, and the surround the complementary responses. All doses of LSD depressed spontaneous neuronal activity. At doses of less than 100 μg, the responses of the center and surround of the receptive fields to photic stimulation were not strongly correlated, suggesting that the drug was influencing the sensory transformation properties of the lateral geniculate nucleus. The authors point out that since the properties of cortical visual neurons are jointly determined by the spontaneous activity and sensory transformation in more peripheral parts of the visual system, the effects of LSD on the lateral geniculate nucleus could at least partly account for the disturbed perceptual experience associated with LSD intake in animals and man (Hoffman and Osmond, 1967).

Not surprisingly, therefore, discriminative behavior is found to be influenced by LSD. In a series of ingenious animal psychophysical experiments, Blough (1957) studied the effect of LSD on a conditional brightness discrimination task in the pigeon. He found improvement in the percentage of correct responses with doses of 200 and 500 µg/kg, which contrasts with some of the later reports of disruptive effects of LSD on certain discrimination tasks. Hearst (1964) subsequently used stimulus generalization methods to demonstrate the specificity of stimulus control in animals before and after the drug. More recently, Brown and Bass (1967) have reported a psychophysical method for training monkeys to make scaling judgments along a size dimension. The letter E was prepared in a constant size and in 3, 5, 10, 15, 20, and 25% size decrements from that constant. Eight monkeys were trained to choose the smaller E from an array of two constants and one comparison stimuli. Failure to select the proper value within 30 seconds or an incorrect choice resulted in a 5-second shock, which could be escaped from by a correct response. LSD in doses as low as 0.1 mg/kg increased reaction times in this task.

Fuster (1959) also found that LSD increased reaction time and decreased accuracy in monkeys responding to tachistoscopically presented objects. Doses of 2 to 8 µg/kg disrupted performance on a cone/pyramid discrimination test presented for 20-msec exposures. Fuster attributed this failure to the demanding level of attention required in the tachistoscopic task, but success depends as much on the accuracy of visual discrimination and quickness of response as on attentiveness. In more recent experiments with monkeys, in which ample time was allowed for attention and response, LSD in doses of 10 to 40 µg/kg disrupted a difficult size discrimination, although an easy one was unaffected. It has been suggested that, in difficult discriminations, even when there is plenty of time to respond, animals shift their attention from relevant to irrelevant dimensions and that LSD facilitates such attentional shifts.

LSD does not impair performance on discriminated avoidance tasks in well-trained rats. This may be because the discrimination part of the task is not taxing to the animals. This would be supported by the observation that initial *acquisition* of discriminated (auditory) avoidance in a pole-jumping situation is impaired in the rat by 50 to 100 µg/kg LSD (Domino et al., 1965). Evarts (1958) found the same to be true of visual discriminations in the highly trained monkey.

Key's 1961 study is one of the few to compare a given dose of LSD in one species on a variety of discrimination tasks. A shock-avoidance task was used in cats trained to cross a 9-in. barrier to avoid a 0.5-ma shock. Three conditions were studied:

1. Sensory generalization. After being trained to cross on presentation of a 600-cps pure tone, the response to tones between 200 and 2000 cps were tested in extinction.

2. Discrimination I. The cat was trained to cross on presentation of a 600-cps tone. Then a 400-cps tone was introduced, and the cat was trained not to cross at that signal.

3. Discrimination II. With two other tones, the cat was again trained to cross to one and not to cross to the other in order to avoid shock. But, in this task, trials on both tones were given from the start of training.

It was found that 15 µg/kg of LSD slowed extinction in the stimulus generalization test, i.e., more responses were made to the conditioned and the generalization stimuli, but the shape of the generalization curve remained the same. Thus, although the animal apparently still discriminated between the stimuli, the significance threshold of auditory signals changed. With discrimination method I, 15 µg/kg of LSD resulted in crossings to both tones, whereas the discrimination trained by Method II remained unaffected. It is suggested that the negative tone in Method I was never very significant to the animal because it was introduced after the conditioned response had been established. With the general increase in stimulus significance induced by LSD, responses to this negative stimulus were shown. By contrast, under Method II, the negative tone was already highly significant to the cat because responses to it had been extinguished. As in other studies, LSD did not affect discriminations based on two highly significant cues in well-trained animals.

In such discrimination experiments, several workers have noted the considerable individual variation of the primate response to LSD. This has also been noted in experiments on more cognitive tasks (Black et al., 1969). Several laboratories have investigated the effect of LSD on delay tasks of various kinds. Evarts (1957) reported that doses as large as 950 µg did not impair delayed response cued by the direct method, i.e., the monkey watches the experimenter hide a peanut reinforcement in one of two spatial locations and then, after a delay, is allowed to retrieve the peanut. If, however, indirect cueing is used, i.e., a discriminative stimulus, such as a form, is presented to indicate where the reinforcement is to be found, then LSD has a much more disruptive effect. In fact, the most severe disruption has been found when indirect delayed response is tested automatically, rather than by a human tester, in the Wisconsin General Test apparatus (WGTA). Black has suggested that a direct-cued DR involves a short-term associative process between reinforcement and position, whereas an indirect-cued DR involves long-term associative processes. LSD apparently affects the lat-

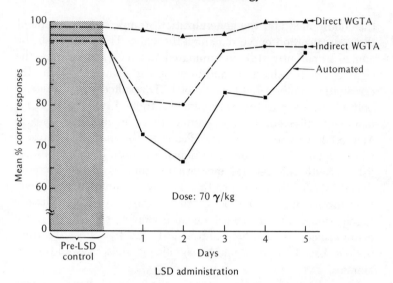

Fig. 4-24 Performance curves on three versions of the delayed response task in a group of four monkeys. At an intermediate dose of LSD, 70 μg/ kg, note the clear differential effect, with impairment occurring in the performance of the indirect and automated tasks and the virtual absence of effect on direct task scores. (Reproduced from Black et al., 1969.)

ter and not the former (Fig. 4-24). Similarly, delayed alternation tested in the automatic WGTA with a 2-second delay was found to be affected by LSD (Jarvik and Chorover, 1960). At some doses, both the accuracy and number of alternation responses were depressed, but at lower doses accuracy, but not response rate, was affected. By contrast, amphetamine and chlorpromazine were found to depress rate but not accuracy. It was suggested that delay tasks are very sensitive to LSD because the drug changes sensitivity to internal and external distracting stimuli. Several workers have noted the rapid development of tolerance to LSD, which is true also in man. It has also been repeatedly noted that the disruptive effects of LSD on discriminative and cognitive tasks persist several weeks after drug administration.

Cannabis

In man, *Cannabis* produces a feeling of well being, improved ideation, and a facilitation of motor activity. After large doses, sense of time and space are eventually lost, and torpor ensues. Animals show a similar combination of depressant and excitatory effects. There is an increase in spontaneous activity, which is hindered by a motor deficit. The animals run around swaying and falling on their sides. These contradictory effects of *Cannabis* are emphasized by the observation that it potentiates both the depressant action of barbiturates and the excitatory action of amphetamine. In early behavioral studies with *Cannabis*, the tendency of the natural compound to decompose when exposed to air made it difficult to evaluate the dose required to produce psychological changes in animals. The synthesis of crystalline Δ^9-THC, the major active component of *Cannabis*, and Δ^8-THC, a minor active component, have been important for the development of animal studies.

The pure compounds Δ^9-THC and Δ^8-THC produce behavior similar to that seen after hallucinogenic drugs are administered in a range of species, and they also disrupt complex behavior involving memory or discrimination. In this respect, *Cannabis* resembles LSD, and, like LSD, it has pronounced effects on the theta wave EEG.

Scheckel et al. (1968) studied the two active cannabinoids in either squirrel or rhesus monkeys trained with operant methods on (a) continuous shock avoidance, (b) titration of shock threshold; and (c) delayed matching of color. On the continuous shock avoidance task, low doses of 4 or 8 mg/kg of Δ^9-THC depressed the avoidance response rate by more than 50%. The monkeys appeared depressed. With higher doses (16-64 mg/kg), the monkeys were highly stimulated, and avoidance responding was often at twice the control rates. The animals were excited and behaved as though they were having visual hallucinations. With 2, 4, and 8 mg/kg Δ^8-THC, stimulation was observed without the depression seen at lower doses. On the Weis and Laties shock titration procedure, 4-8 mg/kg of either compound gave evidence of increased shock tolerance, but it is doubtful if this represents a genuine analgesic effect—the response to shock merely varies more. Delayed matching of color suffered most, being severely disrupted for 4 days by a single dose of 4 mg/kg of Δ^9-THC. In addition to their general depressant or stimulant properties associated with hallucinations, Δ^8- and Δ^9-THC appear to affect high-order cognitive performance most profoundly.

McMillan et al. (1970) reported that the key pecking behavior of piegons performing on a multiple FI/FR schedule was severely depressed by 1.8 mg/kg of Δ^9-THC. The depressant effect is not specific to reinforced behavior, for McMillan (1973a) has shown that on both elements of a multiple FI/FI punishment schedule Δ^9- and Δ^8-THC depress responding. Tolerance to the drug developed rapidly, however, and, after the 5th daily dose, response rates had returned to within the range of the control undrugged rate. The dose of drug was then gradually increased, and, by day 25, a dose of 36 mg/kg rarely depressed responding; indeed, in some sessions, rates of responding were increased. When the drug was stopped, no withdrawal symptoms were observed.

The rapid development of tolerance and the eventual rate-increasing effect of the drug resemble the effects of morphine in pigeons, although, the narcotics do produce strong withdrawal symptoms.

5 | Animal Models and the Neuropharmacological Basis of Nervous and Mental Disorders in Man

In preceding chapters we have reviewed some of the behavioral and neuropharmacological properties of psychoactive drugs. In some instances, it has proved possible to relate the action of a drug on specific aspect of behavior to a plausible neuropharmacological mechanism. Interest in either aspect of the action of psychoactive drugs in animals, however, stems from the need to seek a better understanding of the use of such drugs in man. In this final chapter, a few areas of investigation will be considered in which animal model systems have been developed that may be relevant to an understanding of the neuropharmacology of behavioral disorders in man.

ANIMAL MODELS OF PSYCHOSIS AND THEIR RELEVANCE TO SCHIZOPHRENIA

Schizophrenia is characterized by bizarre thought disorders, disturbance of affect, and withdrawal from meaningful interaction with other people. It is not possible to replicate these conditions in animals by manipulating normal behavioral control. Two lines of evidence, however, have emerged that may lead to an animal analogue of schizophrenia. First, it has been observed that people addicted to amphetamine show a form of psychotic behavior that closely resembles schizophrenia; indeed, not infrequently, amphetamine addicts have been misdiagnosed as paranoid schizophrenics. Second, it has become clear that the neuroleptic drugs that are most useful for alleviating the primary symptoms of schizophrenia act neuropharmacologically as antagonists at CNS dopamine receptors, and a good correlation has been found between their clinical potency and effectiveness and the specificity of their anti-dopaminergic activities.

Amphetamine psychosis in man is characterized by agitation and the ability to verbalize about the abnormal cognitive processes often associated with delusions of persecution. It is known that amphetamine releases both NE and DA in the brain, and it seems probable that the disturbances of response patterns seen in psychosis due to amphetamine abuse are mediated mainly by dopaminergic activity; on the other hand, arousal appears to be controlled by NE systems. If this is the case, then one would predict that a more specific DA-releasing drug or DA receptor agonist drug would produce a psychosis more closely resembling non-paranoid schizophrenia than that induced by amphetamine.

Amphetamine psychosis in human volunteers is conspicuously lacking in thought disorder, although it is possible that the increased level of arousal evoked by the drug masks this symptom. Typically, amphetamine psychosis is associated with delusions, hallucinations in all modalities, and the stereotyped repetition of meaningless patterns of behavior.

If the suggestion of psychological and neuropharmacological similarity between amphetamine psychosis and paranoid schizophrenia is valid, certain further predictions can be made. Mild schizophrenia can be exacerbated by amphetamine administration, and recovered schizophrenics can relapse. The d- and l-isomers of amphetamine, which seem to be pharmacologically equipotent on DA systems, should also be equipotent in inducing psychosis or in influencing the symptoms of schizophrenia; other drugs that increase brain concentrations of free DA should also induce psychosis. All of these predictions have been borne out by experimental work in man. Davis (1974) reports that relapse with the reappearance of hallucinations and delusions can be induced in recovered schizophrenics and that the d- and l-isomers of amphetamine are equipotent in this respect. It is important to note that amphetamine intensifies schizophrenic symptoms, rather than adding different psychotic symptoms to the schizophrenic illness. Patients themselves perceive that their illness is worsening under the influence of the drug. By contrast, when they are treated with LSD, schizophrenics recognize that the psychedelic drug-induced psychosis is of a different character from their own mental disturbance (Janowsky et al. 1973).

Angrist et al. (1971) have compared the ability of the d- and l-isomers of amphetamine to induce central stimulation and psychosis in volunteers who had previously been amphetamine addicts. The two isomers were equipotent in inducing psychosis, but the d-isomer produced much more agitation than the l-isomer. Cocaine is another drug that induces a form of psychosis similar to schizophrenia in man, and, on this basis, it is thought to share the neuropharmacological properties of amphetamine. One interesting anomaly in this pattern of results is the finding that L-dopa, which increases the availability of DA in the brain, fails to induce psychosis. Parkinsonian patients who receive treatment with large doses of L-dopa seldom show any evidence of drug-induced psychosis. But when L-dopa was given to schizophrenic patients an exacerbation of psychosis was observed (Angrist et al., 1973).

Large doses of amphetamine also induce bizarre patterns of behavior in experimental animals, and this offers perhaps the most plausible model for studies of drug-induced "psychosis." Randrup and his collaborators (Randrup and Munkvad, 1970) have made a thorough study of drug-induced "psychosis" in rats and monkeys, and Ellinwood's studies (1972) of "psychosis" in the cat are also noteworthy. In all species, the "psychosis" in many of its features resembles that observed in man. In the rat, a single large dose of amphetamine (10 mg/kg) induces stereotyped behavior. Instead of the normal pattern of locomotion and exploration, the rat exhibits a behavior in which the wide range of normal motor responses is reduced, and a few elements of the behavioral repertoire are repeated continuously. Locomotion and grooming disappear, and rearing, sniffing, licking, and gnawing increase in frequency. The more intense the stereotypy, the fewer the categories of behavior observed, compulsive gnawing being the behavior that predominates in the most intense forms of stereotypy in this species. At this stage, the animal is immobile and may assume highly abnormal postures while it gnaws furiously. There are several reasons for believing that dopaminergic systems are involved in this drug-induced stereotypy. Amphetamine releases NE and DA in the brain, and depletion of these amines by prior treatment with α-methyl tyrosine can completely prevent amphetamine-induced stereotypy. Drugs that block DA receptors (phenothiazines and butyrophenones) also antagonize amphetamine-induced stereotypy, whereas drugs that directly stimulate DA receptors, such as apomorphine, induce stereotypy that is indistinguishable from that produced by amphetamine.

Dopamine is contained in neuronal pathways that project from the regions of the substantia nigra to the basal ganglia and to various parts of the limbic system in the forebrain. Destruction of the substantia nigra or the sites of the DA terminals in the caudate nucleus by surgical means or by administration of 6-hydroxydopamine abolishes amphetamine-induced stereotypy.

Ellinwood et al. (1972) have described in detail the catatonic postures caused by amphetamine in the cat. They refer to dyssynchrony as "a given body ensemble taking an autonomous movement which did not seem to have purpose of relatedness to other body segments." For example, repetitious repositioning or raising movements of the hind legs on many occasions had little or no relation to the sniffing patterns that were taking place at the head and neck. The active front end and the inactive hind end often resulted in a hunchback posture. The cat often appeared to have forgotten where a leg was positioned and left it in an awkward disjunctive position. Other disjunctive postures included uncomfortable sitting and lying positions, very much like those noted in human catatonics. Ellinwood et al. (1972) emphasize the importance of postural attitudinal sets for the normal organization of behavior.

Amphetamine intoxication and schizophrenia in humans are associated with similar patterns of stereotyped behavior and postural dysfunction. In amphetamine psychosis in man, the delusion of skin parasites often results in the emergence of repetitive "grooming" responses. Schizophrenics have abnormal eye movement patterns and spend an unusually large proportion of their time in eye-scan. Amphetamine psychosis is associated with catatonia, and in schizophrenic children and adults postural impairments are often observed.

Other drugs induce excitation and forms of psychosis that differ from that induced by amphetamine. Morphine is one such drug. In rats, small doses of morphine stimulate behavior. Schiørring and Hecht (1974), comparing morphine- and amphetamine-induced excitation in rats, found that amphetamine excitation is associated with a progressive decrease in the number of categories of behavior observed. Initially, locomotion, rearing, and sniffing predominate, but, as the dose increases, locomotion and rearing are not seen and sniffing, licking, and biting emerge. Amphetamine thus disrupts the normal balance of responses, favoring some and inhibiting others. Morphine, by contrast, produces a general excitation, and particular acts do not disappear from the animal's repertoire. It has been noted, however, that self-grooming, particularly with the hind legs, is disproportionately increased by morphine.

The effects of these drugs on social behavior in the rat are also different. Studying pairs of male rats, Silverman (1965) noted that some elements of behavior, such as approaching, following, and mounting, increased, while others, such as sniffing the anogenital region, decreased after amphetamine administration. Using larger groups of rats, Randrup and Munkvad (1970) found that amphetamine in small doses produced abnormal grouping behavior and in larger doses abolished social contact between animals, since individually they were engaged in stereotyped behavior. In monkeys, the social isolation induced by amphetamine is particularly noticeable, since behavioral acts during which animals touch one another, such as grooming, disappear. The effects of morphine on social behavior in grouped rats, however, are markedly different. After administration of 2 mg/kg of morphine, all eight rats in a group performed rapid forward locomotion, rearing, self-grooming, and all normal social behavior elements (grouping, contact sniffing, crawling over and under each other, tactile contact, and following) were present. These behaviors were observed in short, changing sequences. Excited locomotion and quick forward moving with galloping and jumping movements were present during most of the observation period. Thus, unlike amphetamine, morphine induces general stimulation of both individual and social behavior without disruption of behavior patterns.

It is not yet possible to fully understand the significance of these results in animals in relation to the effects of the drugs in human addicts. Both amphetamine and morphine are self-administered in man for their excitatory and euphoric effects, and it is possible that their particular effect on one aspect of behavior rather than another may determine their attractiveness as drugs to different personality types. Schiørring and Hecht (1974) suggested, for example, that the social facilitation induced by morphine may be especially attractive to introverted personalities.

When large doses of morphine are administered to animals, depression rather than the excitation caused by smaller doses is usually observed. If animals are given repeated large doses of morphine, a form of stereotyped behavior may also emerge. Despite its stereotyped nature, the morphine-induced stereotypy is clearly distinguishable from that caused by large doses of amphetamine. Rats indulge in sniffing, licking, and biting of the paws, but this stereotypy is interrupted by bouts of very quick running and standing-up behavior. The neuropharmacological basis of morphine-induced stereotypy is unclear, but it has been proposed that NE, rather than DA, may be predominantly involved (Ayhan and Randrup, 1972).

As pointed out in Chapter 4, it is not easy to characterize the effects of neuroleptic drugs on normal behavior. They are basically depressant, but there is good reason to believe that this behavioral effect may be secondary to some more subtle modulation of behavioral control. This is more than an academic problem for drug companies in search of more effective and specific antipsychotic drugs. A specific battery of animal tests for predicting antipsychotic drugs would be of immense practical importance, and various screening procedures, of course, already exist. Antipsychotic drugs antagonize amphetamine-induced stereotypy strongly, and this fact has provided a useful screening test for evaluating new drugs. Janssen et al. (1965) has described in detail the use of behavioral tests in animals to predict neuroleptic activity. The tests themselves are simple: (a) Drug-induced *catalepsy* and ptosis; (b) antagonism of amphetamine-induced stereotypy; (c) drug effect on shock avoidance in jumping box; (d) antagonism of apomorphine-induced stereotypy; (e) drug alterations of food intake; (f) open-field activity (rearing or ambulation); (g) drug effects on mortality caused by E and NE injections; (h) antagonism of tryptamine-induced limb convulsions; and (i) resistance to rotational trauma. Forty antipsychotic drugs, principally of the phenothiazine and butyrophenone classes, were tested, and an ED_{50} (i.e., the dose of drug producing one-half the maximal response or a specified re-

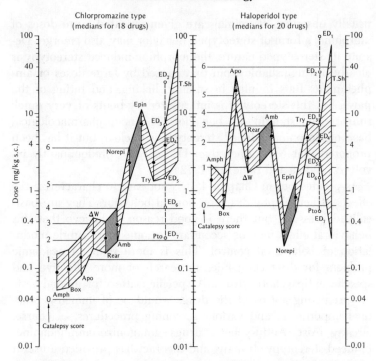

Fig. 5-1 Mean neuroleptic activity spectra of neuroleptic drugs of the haloperidol-type (*left*) and the chlorpromazine-type (*right*)

Amph: ED50	amphetamine test	Amb: ED50	ambulation, open-
Box: ED50	jumping box test		field test
Apo: ED50	apomorphine test	Norepi: ED50	norepinephrine test
ΔW: ED50	ΔW-test, food intake	Epin: ED50	epinephrine test
Rear: ED50	rearing, open-field test	Try: ED50	tryptamine test

The confidence limits ($P = 0.05$) of each ED50 are represented by a vertical line:

Pto: EDx-values, palpebral ptosis test: the lowest open circle represents ED7 the next circle ED6 then ED5 then (black circle) ED4 then ED3 ED2 and ED1

T.Sh.: the vertical line represents the estimated active dose range (lowest active to highest active dose), rotational traumatic shock test.

Catalepsy score: EDx (ED0 to ED6), catalepsy test. The position of each EDx is represented by a horizontal line crossing the entire spectrum.

(Reproduced from Janssen et al., 1965.)

sponse in 50% of animals) was obtained for each test. These values were used to plot "activity spectra," and it was found that the two classes of drug produced clearly distinguishable spectra as illustrated in the mean patterns for all phenothiazines and all butyrophenones (Fig. 5-1).

Neuropharmacological animal model systems have also proved useful for quantifying neuroleptic actions. One unifying hypothesis of the behavioral effects produced by neuroleptic drugs is that they act by blocking DA receptors in the CNS. A recent useful biochemical model for assessing such antagonist actions has come from the finding that neuroleptic drugs block the stimulating effects of DA on cyclic AMP production in homogenates of rat brain striatum or rat mesolimbic nuclei. It has been shown that a series of neuroleptics differed over a 500-fold range in their ability to inhibit the striatal dopamine-sensitive adenylate cyclase.

One complication in the clinical use of the neuroleptic drugs is that they often produce severe extrapyramidal side effects, including a syndrome similar to idiopathic parkinsonism. This syndrome has been explained as a blockade of DA receptors by the drugs, resulting in a functional lack of DA in the basal ganglia. The more potent anti-dopaminergic drugs, however, are used clinically in much lower doses than the less potent drugs, and, on this basis, one might therefore expect all neuroleptics to produce about the same incidence of extrapyramidal signs. That this is not the case has become increasingly apparent. In particular, the phenothiazine, THIORIDAZINE, and the recently described dibenzoazepine, CLOZAPINE, have been shown to produce very few extrapyramidal motor side effects. Recently, Miller and Hiley (1974) have tested the anticholinergic potency of the phenothiazines in a biochemical preparation in which they measured the ability of the drugs to block the binding of a specific receptor label to muscarinic receptors. They found that thioridazine and clozapine were potent anticholinergics, whereas such neuroleptics as FLUPHENAZINE and SPIROPERIDOL, which cause a high incidence of extrapyramidal side effects, were much weaker anticholinergics. Traditionally, the extrapyramidal side effects associated with phenothiazine treatment have been treated by centrally acting anticholinergic agents, which restore the balance between the antagonistic dopaminergic and cholinergic influences in the basal ganglia without interfering with the antipsychotic action of the neuroleptics. These results indicate that the ideal antipsychotic might combine both anticholinergic and anti-dopaminergic activity and that screening procedures combining an anti-muscarinic test with an *in vitro* measure of DA receptor blockade, such as the DA-sensitive adenylate cyclase, may ensure improved and rapid selection of potentially useful neuroleptic drugs.

THE ROLE OF DA IN PARKINSON'S DISEASE

Parkinson's disease is a neurological condition associated with muscular rigidity, a paucity of voluntary movements (akinesia), and tremor. It is progressive and seriously debilitating. It has long been known to be associated with neuropathological changes in the basal ganglia. Several different forms and etiologies of the disease have been recognized. In cases where tremor is the dominant symptom, patients have often been treated by the surgical production of lesions in certain thalamic nuclei associated with motor control and thought to be involved in the maintenance of the abnormal tremor. The rigidity and akinesia symptoms that predominate in other groups of patients have been treated with drugs, and anticholinergics were known to alleviate the symptoms long before the neuropharmacological rationale of this therapy was appreciated. When the distribution of amine transmitters in the brain was described, it became apparent that the basal ganglia had a rich dopaminergic innervation, and biochemical analysis of post-mortem parkinsonian brain tissue revealed abnormally low levels of DA and tyrosine hydroxylase in the caudate nucleus and other regions of the neostriatum. This biochemical defect, together with evidence of cell loss from the substantia nigra, the site of origin of the dopaminergic nigro-striatal system, confirmed the neurochemical basis of at least the rigidity and akinesia symptoms in Parkinson's disease.

These findings resulted in the development of a new pharmacological treatment for parkinsonism. It was argued that, since the disease was associated with a deficiency of DA in the brain, biochemical manipulations that temporarily replenished DA stores should improve the extrapyramidal motor symptoms. But DA itself could not be given, since it would not pass the blood-brain barrier. It was found, however, that l-dopa, an aminoacid precursor of DA, did enter the brain to increase brain DA in experimental animals. l-Dopa therapy for parkinsonism was introduced and proved highly successful. This represents the first example of the rational development of a drug treatment for a CNS disorder based on a neurochemical understanding of the nature of the disease. As far as the rigidity and akinesia symptoms are concerned, l- dopa has revolutionized the prognosis for many parkinsonian patients. The improvement in motor performance is rapid, once l-dopa treatment is started, and bedridden patients can often resume normal activities.

The neurochemical coordination of basal ganglia structures has been further explored in animal preparations. It appears that the synthesis of DA in the nigro-striatal pathway is controlled partly by a feedback loop from the striatum to the substantia nigra, and ACh is thought to be the transmitter at the regulating synapses. In addition, there is a strong cholinergic input to the striatum itself, and the fact that anti-cholinergic drugs are used successfully to treat parkinsonism suggests that there is a cholinergic/dopaminergic balance involved in the normal control of motor function.

Animal model systems have been devised to study anti-parkinsonian drugs. The apparently simple neurological and neurochemical basis of Parkinson's disease encouraged attempts to produce a similar defect in animals by the placement of lesions in the nigro-striatal system. Such lesions in rats, cats, and monkeys, however, disrupt normal motor behavior but do not closely mimic the clinical syndrome. This is perhaps not surprising. Parkinson's disease develops in patients over a period of many years, and such a gradual eroding of neural substrates may well induce subtle adaptive changes in nervous functions that cannot be mimicked by a sudden experimental assault on the same structure. Larochelle et al. (1971) have pursued this problem in both cats and monkeys. Although discrete substantia nigra lesions in the monkey did not produce parkinsonian symptoms, more extensive extrapyramidal damage involving the substantia nigra and the neural circuit between the red nucleus and the cerebellum induced tremor. Damage to the latter circuit plus treatment with the MAO inhibitor, harmaline, produced the same effect. In monkeys with the combination lesions, L-dopa treatment markedly improved the motor disturbances.

Bilateral substantia nigra lesions, therefore, do not produce an animal model of Parkinson's disease. Ungerstedt (1971), however, has developed a unilateral substantia nigra lesion preparation that has proved useful in evaluating drugs that influence the dopaminergic functioning of the basal ganglia.

The lesion was made by injecting 6-OHDA through a cannula placed in the substantia nigra to selectively destroy amine-containing neurons, in this case, the nigro-striatal DA pathway; widespread non-specific damage to nearby systems was thus avoided. After the immediate postoperative effects on motor behavior have subsided, the rats show circling motor activity if the dopaminergic system is stimulated pharmacologically. The rats are placed in a circular dome to provide an easy way of constraining circling, and a recording mechanism attached to

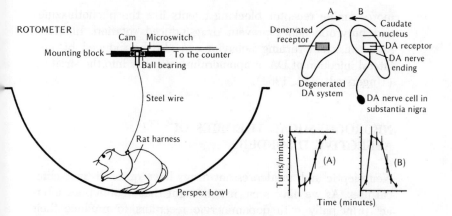

Fig. 5-2 *Left:* A schematic drawing of the rotometer. The movements of the rat are transferred by the steel wire to the microswitch arrangement. *Upper right:* the principal outline of the experimental situation shown in a horizontal projection of the negro-striatal DA system. When stimulation of the denervated receptor dominates, the animals rotates in direction A. When stimulation of the innervated receptor dominates, the animal rotates in direction B. *Lower right:* the rotational behavior is presented as turns per minute versus time. The curves are given negative y-values when stimulation of the denervated receptor dominates and positive y-values when stimulation of the innervated receptor dominates. Each point represents the mean ($\pm$ S.E.M.) of a certain number of animals. (Reproduced from Ungerstedt, 1971.)

the back of the rat automatically cumulates rotations. In this so-called "ROTOMETER," drugs that release amines (e.g., amphetamine, cocaine) produce turning toward the side of the lesion, whereas DA agonists (e.g., apomorphine, L-dopa) produce turning in the opposite direction (Fig. 5-2). It is suggested that the nigro-striatal degeneration results in the loss of presynaptic DA and postsynaptic supersensitivity on the side of the lesion. Therefore, drugs that release amines have less influence on this side of the basal ganglia, whereas receptor stimulators have more. Amine receptor blocking agents like the phenothiazines and butyrophenones prevent drug-induced rotation. In intact rats, consistent turning behavior can also be induced by unilateral injection of DA or apomorphine directly into the striatum (Ungerstedt et al., 1969).

NEUROCHEMICAL THEORIES OF AFFECTIVE DISORDERS

Neuroleptic and antidepressant drugs have quite distinct clinical uses. As we have seen, it is thought that neuroleptics interact principally with dopaminergic receptors to produce their antipsychotic effects. In contrast, antidepressants are used to relieve behavioral disorders associated with changes in mood. Although they are difficult to dissociate from neuroleptics by any simple animal behavioral parameter, the antidepressants can be clearly distinguished by their neuropharmacological properties. Antidepressants are potent inhibitors of NE and 5-HT uptake sites in the brain, resulting in an increase in the availability of NE and 5-HT at CNS receptors, and this neurochemical effect is thought to underlie their therapeutic action. It has, therefore, been reasoned that NE and/or 5-HT may be involved in the behavioral disorder seen in depression and that the illness may be associated with a reduced availability or release of these amine transmitters.

Depression has not been adequately characterized, behaviorally, but insensitivity to reinforcement has been suggested as a core symptom. There is growing evidence that activity in NE-containing neuronal systems occurs during response to events of affective significance. Reinforcement is an important class of such events, and it induces emotional responses in animals and man. The activity of noradrenergic sympathetic neurons in the periphery is correlated with emotional state and so too is noradrenergic activity in the forebrain. Norepinephrine-containing neurons in the pons and medulla have fibers that project in the medial forebrain bundle to innervate the cortex, limbic system, and hypothalamus. Emotional responses involve both general arousal and response to a particular stimulus complex, and there is reason to suppose that NE is involved in both processes. Amphetamine, for example, is thought to induce somatomotor arousal by releasing NE in the forebrain.

Intracranial self-stimulation has proved to be a valuable technique for studying the pharmacological properties of reinforcement processes. Animals will respond to obtain electric stimulation of various brain areas, and this behavior has all the characteristics of that maintained by such natural reinforcers as food and water. It, therefore, provides a convenient way of determining, experimentally, whether an animal is responsive to reinforcing events. In line with the noradrenergic theory of reinforcement is the observation that the placement of electrodes in the medial forebrain bundle, which contains NE fibers, sustains the highest rates of intracranial self-stimulation. If the synthesis of catecholamines is blocked with α-methyl tyrosine, or if catecholamine receptors are blocked with chlorpromazine, intracranial self-stimulation behavior is abolished.

The importance of NE over DA was stressed by Wise and Stein (1969), who abolished self-stimulation behavior with disulfiram, an inhibitor that prevents the synthesis of NE from DA but leaves brain NE unaffected. Intraventricular l-NE reinstated self-stimulation behavior in such animals, whereas DA and 5-HT did not. It is possible that NE is released from terminals in the hypothalamus and limbic system in response to reinforcing events. Responses to unpleasant events also appear to influence NE activity. Shock avoidance in rats is dependent on brain content of NE; induced fighting behavior or social aggregation increase the rate of turnover of NE in the brain, as does repetitive foot shock.

In clinical studies, a correlate has been found between endogenous amine levels and some aspects of depression and

TABLE 5-1
DRUGS AFFECTING BRAIN NOREPINEPHRINE AND DEPRESSIVE BEHAVIOR

Drug	Behavior (human)	Behavior (animal)	Effect in brain	Suggested mechanism of action
Imipramine-type drugs: Imipramine, desipramine, amitriptyline, desmethylamitriptyline	Effective antidepressant in humans	Prevents reserpine-induced depression in animals	Functional NE potentiation	Blocks re-uptake of NE by axonal membrane
Monoamine oxidase inhibitors	Effective antidepressant	Prevents reserpine-induced depression in animals	Increases NE in many species	Blocks intracellular deamination of NE by MAO
Reserpine	Depression in some humans	Depresses activity (reserpine model of depression)	Depletes NE	Interferes with NE storage in cell—possibly by interfering with uptake and release in storage granules
Methyldopa	Depression in some humans	Depresses activity	Depletes NE	Methyldopa metabolites deplete NE from storage granule

(Reproduced from Bunney and Davis, 1965.)

mania (Bunney and Davis, 1965). It has been observed that certain drugs that lower brain catecholamine and 5-HT levels commonly result in depression as a side effect (Table 5-1). For example, reserpine and tetrabenazine, which have been used to treat hypertension in man, are reported to produce depression in a small but consistent percentage of cases, whereas most other antihypertensive drugs do not have this effect. These cases of reserpine depression are clinically similar to endogenous depression; suicidal tendencies are present, and the depression responds to electroconvulsive therapy. In animals, these drugs also induce a marked depression of ongoing behavior and are shown to deplete brain stores of monoamines severely. Other drugs that deplete endogenous transmitters have been investigated for their tendency to induce depression, pursuant to a "biogenic amine" theory of depression. The antihypertensive, guanethidine, does not penetrate the blood-brain barrier and does not produce depression. By contrast, methyldopa, which is also used as an antihypertensive, and which does enter the brain, is reported to induce depression.

The correlation between brain amines and depression has so far been inferred on the basis of neurochemical studies in animals and clinical observations in man. But in several centers, attempts have been made to obtain neurochemical data in depressed patients. Clearly, brain transmitter levels cannot be measured, but the amount of catecholamine metabolites excreted in the urine has been used as an index of the rate of release of endogenous transmitters. But urinary catecholamine metabolites must primarily reflect activity of peripheral rather than CNS noradrenergic mechanisms. One must, therefore, be cautious in interpreting reports of increased normetanephrine excretion in manic depressive patients and decreased urinary normetanephrine and 3-methoxy, 4-hydroxymandelic acid excretion in these patients during treatment with such antidepressive drugs as imipramine (Schildkraut, 1965). A more direct approach is to measure the concentrations of catecholamines,

5-HT, and their metabolites in samples of cerebrospinal fluid (CSF). Several groups have undertaken such investigations, and most—but not all—have found unusually low concentrations of the 5-HT metabolite 5-hydroxyindoleacetic acid (5-HIAA) in CSF from depressed patients. There is little change in 5-HIAA concentration in CSF in depressed patients after clinical recovery, however, suggesting that the abnormality of 5-HT metabolism may not be related directly to the clinical state. The catecholamine metabolites in CSF have also been investigated, but here there is far less agreement among investigators. The main NE metabolite, 3-methoxy,4-hydroxyphenyl glycol, has been found to be normal in some studies but abnormally low in others. An even more direct approach has been to examine the concentrations of amines in brain tissue obtained post-mortem. Several studies have shown an abnormally low concentration of 5-HT in brain tissue from depressed patients who committed suicide. Taken together, the clinical biochemical studies so far lend more support to the notion that depression is associated with a deficiency of 5-HT rather than with NE systems in the brain (see Coppen, 1974). This view is also supported by the fact that antidepressant drugs of both the MAO inhibitor and tricyclic type affect 5-HT metabolism and uptake greatly. The amino acid precursor for 5-HT synthesis, L-tryptophan, has also been found to increase the antidepressant action of MAO inhibitors in some patients, whereas L-dopa does not.

MODEL SYSTEMS OF ADDICTION

Many psychoactive drugs are self-administered by otherwise normal people because of their ability to induce pleasurable changes in perception and affect. Commonly abused drugs include arousal-changing drugs such as the amphetamines and barbiturates, mood-changing drugs such as the opiates, and hallucinogenic drugs such as lysergic acid derivatives and *Cannabis.*

As described previously (Chapter 2), not all such drugs cause tolerance or addiction, although these phenomena tend to occur with the barbiturates, amphetamines, and opiates. A hazard associated with the development of tolerance is that as the dosage is progressively increased, it may reach levels at which the drug is generally toxic as well as psychoactive. In addition to tolerance, physical dependence is seen with some of the drugs of abuse. Dependence is associated with a physiological craving and need for the drug, and withdrawal of the drug results in intense physical discomfort.

Once dependence has developed, the withdrawal syndrome cannot be avoided if the addiction is to be overcome, although the physical discomfort can be alleviated during withdrawal—for example, by treatment with some other less active analogue of the addictive drug, such as methadone.

Although the development of pharmacological tools, such as methadone, for controlling addiction are important, there has recently been a growing interest in studying the behavioral basis of drug addiction. Why are drugs reinforcing? Are some aspects of the drug-taking habit, in addition to the physiological aspect, reinforcing? If so, can behavioral therapy be used to overcome addiction? These questions can only be answered by well-designed experiments, and, for this reason, studies of the self-administration of drugs by animals are important. Most relevant to the human situation seem to be monkey addicts, and with these animals it has been possible to begin to demonstrate the nature of the behavioral control exerted by drugs and the properties of tolerance, dependence, and withdrawal, properties that are so germane to the human addiction problem.

The experiments of Thompson and Pickens (1971) are noteworthy in this area. They have compared various routes of self-administration of a wide range of addictive drugs in both monkeys and rats. The appropriate route of administration varies with the drug; cocaine and morphine are self-administered through intravenous jugular vein catheters, whereas alcohol is administered orally and *Cannibis* by inhalation of its smoke. An important general finding is that drugs control behavior in precisely the same way as do traditional reinforcers. Fixed-ratio, fixed-interval, and variable-interval schedules of drug reinforcement generate response patterns that are indistinguishable from those maintained by food, water, or shock avoidance. Deprivation, satiation, and the size of the reinforcement (i.e., dose of drug) used all influence responding in a predictable manner.

There are various pitfalls with this research, but they can be overcome. For example, how does one initially encourage a monkey to self-administer drugs orally? A behavioral phenomenon called "psychogenic polydipsia" is utilized to achieve this end. Rats, if rewarded with dry food on a variable-interval schedule, drink abnormally large quantities of water. Once a high fluid intake is established in this way, drug-adulterated drink is provided, and self-administration is established quite rapidly. This method has been used for alcohol, and morphine intake has also been induced in this way. This research is also complicated by the fact that drugs often have an immediate effect on behavior, influencing the pattern of responding quite independently from their reinforcing action. Periods of extinction after reinforcement circumvent this problem; the periods can be varied depending upon how long the drug effect lasts, or multiple schedules can be used with food and drug reinforcement alternating. Any general depressant or excitatory effect of the drug would influence behavior controlled with either reinforcer and could thus be distinguished from effects specific to drug-reinforced behavior.

Self-administration techniques, in addition to providing a convenient way of demonstrating the reinforcing properties of drugs, can also be used in model systems to investigate addictive behavior. Self-administration of alcohol provides one such example. Winger and Woods (1973) implanted rhesus monkeys with jugular vein catheters and gave them continuous access to a lever that initiated injections of 15% w/v ethanol. Under these conditions, monkeys became intoxicated. Of particular interest is the observation that response rates for alcohol do not escalate as has been observed in self-administration studies with such other drugs of dependence as morphine or barbiturates. Voluntary abstinence is another unique feature of alcohol self-administration. Monkeys take in large quantities of alcohol and then stop responding for some time, whereupon withdrawal symptoms are observed. This pattern of behavior has been likened to that in the human "binge" drinker, and serves a useful function because alcohol is toxic in large doses, and continual intake might quickly lead to death. It is suggested that after a large dose of alcohol these toxic effects override any reinforcing property of the drug and inhibit further intake. Similar patterns of "self-abstinence" have been observed in humans under experimental conditions (Mello and Mendelson, 1972).

Self-administration techniques with monkeys are used to demonstrate the disruptive effect of withdrawal symptoms on ongoing behavior. Withdrawal can either be initiated by abstinence (Thompson and Schuster, 1964) or by the use of such morphine antagonists as nalorphine or naloxone. Goldberg et al. (1971) have shown that both antagonists severely disrupt ongoing behavior in morphine-dependent monkeys. It has subsequently been demonstrated that in such monkeys the antagonists act as aversive stimuli, and animals will learn to respond to avoid injections of these compounds (Goldberg et al., 1972). Further evidence that withdrawal is aversive and disrupts behavior is afforded by the studies of Holtzman and Villareal (1973), in which monkeys worked for food on a multiple VI/VI punishment schedule. Chronic morphine treatment depressed behavior on both segments of the schedule. Although withdrawal of morphine did not affect depressed responding on the VI food part of the schedule, responding during punishment was paradoxically greatly increased. It is proposed by Holtzman and Villareal

(1973) that "the increases in punished responding suggest that disinhibition of behavior under punishment control may be a factor in the antisocial behavior of human addicts undergoing withdrawal from narcotic analgesics."

In our discussion of the behavioral effects of morphine (Chapter 4), experiments were described to demonstrate that conditioned stimuli associated with narcotic injections can reverse withdrawal and maintain drug-seeking behavior in the absence of drug reinforcement. It has been shown in morphine-dependent monkeys and rats that conditioned stimuli associated with withdrawal symptoms can themselves elicit physiological disturbances characteristic of those following narcotic withdrawal (see Chapter 4, pp. 219-222). These observations have been verified and extended in a recent study (Drawburgh and Lal, 1974). Rats were made morphine-dependent by injections in the presence of a ball. A 24-hour withdrawal induced a hypothermic response, which was reversed if the ball was presented. Naloxone, a morphine antagonist, also induced withdrawal hypothermia, but presentation of the ball did not reverse this effect. The fact that naloxone blocks the psychological responses evoked by conditioned stimuli in the same way it blocks the unconditioned morphine effects has both theoretical and practical implications. Of theoretical importance is the suggestion that the conditional stimulus may evoke activity in the brain pathways specifically sensitive to the agonistic actions of morphine and to morphine dependence. The practical importance of this finding is related to the use of narcotic antagonists in the therapy of narcotic addiction. The current rationale behind the use of narcotic antagonists in the treatment of heroin addicts is that these drugs extinguish heroin consumption because they block the "high" sought from the agonist effects of the drug. Since narcotic antagonists appear to block the effects of conditioned stimuli associated with drug intake, as well as the response to the drug itself, they may be valuable in extinguishing a morphine habit associated with the conditional placebo effects of

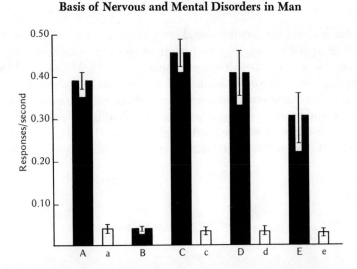

Fig. 5-3 Responses during amphetamine reinforcement, extinction, and amphetamine priming. Columns shown in black (A, B, C, D, and E) refer to the mean (± S.E.) rates of responding during those periods of experimental sessions in which response-contingent infusions of either the drug or saline were available; columns shown in white (a, c, d, and e) refer to mean (± S.E.) rates of responding recorded during time-out (TO). Column A refers to phase 1 (response-contingent infusions of amphetamine); column B to phase 2 (extinction). Columns C, D, and E refer to rates of responding (mean ± S.E.) following amphetamine pretreatment at doses of 1.00 mg/kg (C), 0.30 mg/kg (D), and 0.15 mg/kg (E), respectively. (Reproduced from Stretch and Gerber, 1973.)

morphine-seeking behavior. These effects have been considered to be major factors in "cured" morphine addicts who go back to morphine use.

Insofar as the stimuli associated with drug intake can influence similar behavior at a different time, drug-seeking behavior may be considered "state-dependent." Stretch and Gerber's (1973) study of amphetamine self-administration in the monkey supports this consideration. Monkeys were trained on progressive ratio schedule (i.e., increasing number of responses per reinforcement) for infusions of d-amphetamine (Fig. 5-3, column A). Responding was then extinguished by saline injections (Fig. 5-3, column B). At this stage, amphetamine (1.0, 0.30, or 0.15 mg/kg) was infused 1 minute before the start of a session, and saline injections were continued throughout the sessions. Under these conditions, responses on the FR schedule re-emerge and reach the level associated with amphetamine reinforcements in the first part of the experiment (Fig. 5-3, columns C, D, and E).

References

Aghajanian, G. K. (1975). *In Handbook of Psychopharmacology* (L. Iversen, S. Iversen, and S. Snyder, eds.). vol. 3. New York: Plenum.

Aghajanian, G. K., W. E. Foote, and M. H. Sheard (1970). Action of psychotogenic drugs on single midbrain raphe neurones. J. Pharmac. exp. Ther. 171:178-87.

Angrist, B. M., G. Sathananthan, and S. Gershon (1973). Behavioural effects of L-DOPA in schizophrenic patients. Psychoph. 31:1-12.

Angrist, B. M., B. Shopsin, and S. Gershon (1971). The comparative psychotomimetic effects of stereoisomers of amphetamine. Nature 234: 152-54.

Ayhan, I. H. and A. Randrup (1972). Role of brain noradrenaline in morphine-induced stereotyped behaviour. Psychopharmacologia (Berl.) 27:203-12.

Azrin, N. H. (1956). Some effects of two intermittent schedules of immediate and non-immediate punishment. J. Psychol. 42:3-21.

Azrin, N. H. (1958). Some effects of noise on human behavior. J. exp. anal. Behav. 1:183-200.

Azrin, N. H. and W. C. Holtz (1966). Punishment. In *Operant Behavior: Areas of Research and Application* (W. K. Honig, ed.). New York: Appleton-Century-Crofts, pp. 300-447.

Azrin, N. H., W. C. Holtz, and D. F. Hake (1963). Fixed-ratio punishment. J. exp. anal. Behav. 6:141-48.

Azrin, N. H., R. R. Hutchinson, and D. F. Hake (1966). Extinction-induced aggression. J. exp. anal. Behav. 9:191-204.

Azrin, N. H., R. R. Hutchinson, and R. McLaughlin (1965). The opportunity for aggression as on operant reinforcer during aversive stimulation. J. exp. anal. Behav. 8:171-80.

Baltzer, V. and L. Weiskrantz (1970). Negative and positive behavioural contrast in the same animals. Nature 228:581-82.

Barfield, R. J. and B. D. Sachs (1968). Sexual behavior: Stimulation by painful electric shock to the skin in male rats. Science, 161:393-95.

References

Barondes, S. H. and H. D. Cohen (1968). Memory impairment after subcutaneous injection of aceloxycyloheximide. Science 160, 556-557.

Bender, L. (1947). Childhood schizophrenia. Amer. J. Orthopsychiat. 17: 40-56.

Berger, B. D. and L. Stein (1969). An analysis of the learning deficits produced by scopolamine. Psychopharmacologia (Berl.) 14:271-83.

Berlyne, D. E. (1955). The arousal and satiation of perceptual curiosity in the rat. J. comp. physiol. Psychol. 48:238-46.

Björklund, A., B. Falck and U. Stenevi (1970). On the possible existence of a new interneuronal monoamine in the spinal cord of the rat. J. Pharmac. exp. Ther. 175:525-32.

Black, P., S. N. Cianci, P. Spyropoulos, and J. D. Maser (1969). Behavioral effects of LSD in subhuman primates. In Drugs and the Brain. (P. Black, ed.). Baltimore: Johns Hopkins Press, pp. 291-99.

Bleuler, E. (1911). Dementia Praecox or the Group of Schizophrenias. New York: International University Press. (English trans. by J. Zinkin, 1950.)

Blough, D. S. (1957). Some effects of drugs on visual discrimination in the pigeon. Ann. N.Y. Acad. Sci 66:733-39.

Bradley, P. B. (1968). Synaptic transmission in the central nervous system and its relevance for drug action. Int. Rev. Neurobiol. 11:1-56.

Bradley, P. B. and J. Elkes (1957). The effects of some drugs on the electrical activity of the brain. Brain 80:77-117.

Brady, J. V. (1958). Ulcers in "executive" monkeys. Scient. Amer. 199: 95-100.

Bridges, K. M. B. (1932). Emotional development in early infancy. Child Develop. 3:324-41.

Broadhurst, P. (1961). Abnormal animal behaviour. In Handbook of Abnormal Psychology. (H. J. Eysenck, ed.). New York: Basic Books, pp. 726-63.

Bronson, G. W. (1968). The development of fear in man and other animals. Child Develop. 39:409-31.

Brown, H. and W. C. Bass (1967). Effect of drugs on visually controlled avoidance behavior in rhesus monkeys: A psychophysical analysis. Psychopharmacologia (Berl.) 11:142-53.

Bunney, B. and G. Aghajanian (1974). In Frontiers in Catecholamine Research. (E. Usdin & S. Snyder, eds.). Oxford: Pergamon.

Bunney, W. E. and J. M. Davis (1965). Norepinephrine in depressive reactions. Arch. Gen. Psychiat. 13:483-94.

Bunney, B. S., G. K. Aghajanian, and R. H. Roth (1973). Nature (New Biology) 245:123-25.

Carlsson, S. G. (1972). Effects of apomorphine on exploration. Phys. & Behav. 9:127-29.

References

Carlton, P. L. (1963). Cholinergic mechanism in the control of behaviour by the brain. Psychol. Rev. **70**:19-39.

Chance, M. R. A. and A. P. Silverman (1964). The structure of social behaviour and drug action. In *Animal Behaviour and Drug Action*. Ciba Foundation Symposium. London: J and A Churchill Ltd., pp. 65-79.

Cherek, D. R., T. Thompson, and G. T. Heistad (1973). Responding maintained by the opportunity to attack during an interval food reinforcement schedule. J. exp. anal. Behav. **19**:113-24.

Clark, F. C. and B. J. Steele (1966). Effects of d-amphetamine on performance under a multiple schedule in the rat. Psychopharmacologia (Berl.) **9**:157-69.

Cook, L., A. Davidson, D. J. Davis, and R. T. Kelleher (1960). Epinephrine, norepinephrine, and acetylcholine as conditioned stimuli for avoidance behavior. Science **131**:990-91.

Cook, L. and R. T. Kelleher (1962). Drug effects on the behavior of animals. N.Y. Acad. Sci. **96**:315-35.

Cook, L. and R. T. Kelleher (1963). Effects of drugs on behaviour. Ann. Rev. Pharm. **3**:205-22.

Coppen, A. (1974). In *Biochemistry and Mental Illness*. S. Rose and L. Iversen, eds.). London: Biochem. Society Publications. (in press).

Courvoisier, S., J. Fournel, R. Ducrot, M. Kolsky, and P. Koetschet (1953). Propriétés pharmacodynamiques du chlorhydrate de Chloro-3 (Dieméthylamino-3-propyl)-10 phénothiazines (4.560 R. P.) Arch. intern. Pharmacodynamie **92**:305-61.

Crespi, L. P. (1944). Amount of reinforcement and level of performance. Psychol. Rev. **51**:341-57.

Dahlström, A. and K. Fuxe (1964). A method for the demonstration of monoamine containing nerve fibres in the central nervous system. Acta. physiol. Scand. **60**:293-95.

Davenport, R. K. and E. W. Menzel (1963). Stereotyped behaviour of the infant chimpanzee. Arch. Gen. Psychiat. **8**:99-104.

Davis, J. M. (1974). In *Frontiers in Catecholamine Research*. (E. Usdin and S. H. Snyder, eds.). Oxford: Pergamon.

Deutsch, J. A. (1971). The cholinergic synapse and the site of memory. Science **174**:788-94.

de Wied, D. (1974). Pituitary-adrenal system hormones and behavior. In *The Neurosciences, Third Study Program*. (F. O. Schmitt and F. G. Worden, eds.). Cambridge (Mass.): MIT Press, pp. 653-66.

Dews, P. B. (1955a). Studies on behavior. I. Differential sensitivity to pentobarbital of pecking performance in pigeons depending on the schedule of reward. J. Pharmac. exp. Ther. **113**:393-401.

Dews, P. B. (1955b). Studies on behavior. II. The effects of pentobarbital, methamphetamine and scopolamine on performance in

References

pigeons involving discriminations. J. Pharmac. exp. Ther. **115**:380-89.

Dews, P. B. (1958). Studies on behaviour. IV. Stimulant actions of methamphetamine. J. Pharmac. exp. Ther. **122**:137-47.

Dews, P. B. (1964). A behavioural effect of amobarbital. N-S Arch. Exp. Path. u. Pharmak. **248**:296-307.

Dews, P. B. and W. H. Morse (1961). Behavioural pharmacology. Ann. Rev. Pharm. **1**:145-74.

Dinsmoor, J. A. (1952). A discrimination based on punishment. Quart. J. exp. Psychol. **4**:27-45.

Domino, E. F., A. J. Karoly, and E. L. Walker (1958). Differential effects of some CNS depressants on a quantitative shock avoidance response in the dog. J. Pharmac. exp. Ther. **122**:20 A.

Domino, E. F., D. F. Caldwell, and R. Henke (1965). Effects of psychoactive agents on acquisition of conditioned pole jumping in rats. Psychopharmacologia (Berl.) **8**:285-89.

Drawbaugh, R. and H. Lal (1974). Reversal by narcotic antagonist of a narcotic action elicited by a conditioned stimulus. Nature **247**:65-67.

Ellinwood, E. H., A. Sudilovsky, and L. Nelson (1972) Behavioral analysis of chronic amphetamine intoxication. Biol. Psychol. **4**:215-30.

Emley, G. S. and R. R. Hutchinson (1972). Basis of behavioral influence of chlorpromazine. Life Sciences **11**:43-47.

Estes, W. K. (1944). An experimental study of punishment. Psychol. Monographs **57**:1-40.

Estes, W. K. and Skinner, B. F. (1941). Some quantitative properties of anxiety. J. exp. Psychol. **29**:390-400.

Evarts, E. V. (1957). A review of the neurophysiological effects of lysergic acid diethylamide (LSD) and other psychomimetic agents. Ann. N.Y. Acad. Sci. **66**:479-95.

Evarts, E. V. (1958). Neurophysiological correlates of pharmacologically-induced behavioral disturbances. Proc. Ann. Res. Nerv. Ment. Dis. **36**:347-80.

Falk, J. L. (1972). The nature and determinants of adjunctive behavior. In *Schedule effects: Drugs, Drinking and Aggression.* (R. M. Gilbert and J. D. Keehn, eds.). Toronto: University of Toronto Press.

Fantz, R. L. (1964). Visual experience in infants: Decreased attention to familiar patterns relative to novel ones. Science **146**:668-70.

Feldman, R. S. (1964). Further studies on assay and testing of fixation-preventing psychotropic drugs. Psychopharmacologia (Berl.) **6**:130-42.

Feldman, R. S. and K. F. Green (1966). Effects of chlordiazepoxide on fixated behavior in squirrel monkeys. J. Psychopharm. **1**:37-45.

Ferster, C. B. (1966). Animal behavior and mental illness. Psychol. Rec. **16**:345-56.

Findley, J. D. (1966). Programmed environments for the experimental

References

analysis of human behavior. In *Operant behavior: Areas of Research and Application.* (W. K. Honig, ed.). New York: Appleton-Century Crofts, pp. 827-43.

Flexner, L. B., J. B. Flexner, and R. B. Roberts (1967). Memory in mice analyzed with antibiotics, Science 155:1377-83.

Fuster, J. M. (1959). Lysergic acid and its effects on visual discrimination in monkeys. J. Nerv. Ment. Dis. 129:252-56.

Garcia, J. and R. A. Koelling (1966). Relation of cue to consequence in avoidance learning. Psychon. Sci. 4:123-24.

Geller, I. (1962). Use of approach avoidance behavior (conflict) for evaluating depressant drugs. In *Sixth Hannemann Symposium on Psychosomatic Medium.* (Nadine, ed.). Chap. 33.

Geller, I. and J. Seifter (1960). The effects of meprobromate, barbiturates, d-amphetamine and promazine on experimentally induced conflict in the rat. Psychopharmacologia. 1:482-92.

Geller, I., E. Backman and J. Seifter (1963). Effects of reserpine and morphine on behaviour suppressed by punishment. Life Sciences 4: 226-31.

Geller, I., J. T. Kulak, and J. Seifter (1962). The effects of chlordiazepoxide and chlorpromazine on a punishment discrimination. Psychopharmacologia (Berl.) 25:112-16.

Gendreau, P., D. Sherlock, T. Parsons, R. McLean, G. D. Scott, and M. D. Suboski (1972). Effects of methamphetamine on well-practiced discrimination conditioning of the eyelid response. Psychopharmacologia (Berl.) 25:112-16.

Glaser, D. C. (1910). The formation of habits at high speed. J. comp. Neur. 20:165-84.

Glick, S. D. and M. E. Jarvik (1969). Impairment by d-amphetamine of delayed performance in monkeys. J. Pharmac. exp. Ther. 169:1-6.

Goldberg, S. R. and C. R. Schuster (1967). Conditioned suppression by a stimulus associated with nalorphine in morphine-dependent monkeys. J. exp. anal. Behav. 10:235-42.

Goldberg, S. R., J. H. Woods, and C. R. Schuster (1971). Nalorphine-induced changes in morphine self-administration in rhesus monkeys. J. Pharmac. exp. Ther. 176:464-71.

Goldberg, S. R., F. Hoffmeister, U. Schlichting, and W. Nuttke (1972). Aversive properties of nalorphine and naloxone in morphine-dependent rhesus monkeys. J. Pharmac. exp. Ther. 179:268-76.

Goldstein, A. and P. Sheehan (1969). Tolerance to opioid narcotics. 1. Tolerance to the "running fit" caused by levorphanol in the mouse. J. Pharmac. exp. Ther. 169:175-84.

Goldstein, A., L. Aranow, and S. M. Kalman (1969). In *Principles of Drug Action.* New York: Harper & Row.

References

Green, D. and D. Grahame-Smith (1975). In *Handbook of Psychopharmacology.* (L. Iversen, S. Iversen, and S. Snyder, eds.). vol. 1. New York: Plenum.

Groh, G. and M. Lemieuz (1968). The effect of LSD-25 on spider web formation. Int. J. Addictions 3:41-53.

Hanson, H. M., J. J. Witoslawski, E. H. Campbell, and A. G. Itkin (1966). Estimation of relative antiavoidance activity of depressant drugs in squirrel monkeys. Arch. intern. Pharmacodynamie 161:7-16.

Harlow, H. F. and M. K. Harlow (1965). The affectional systems. In *Behaviour of Non-human Primates.* (A. M. Schrier, H. F. Harlow, and F. Stollnitz, eds.). vol. 2. New York: Academic Press.

Hearst. E. (1964). Drug effects on stimulus generalization gradients in monkeys. Psychopharmacologia (Berl.). 6:57-70.

Hearst, E., M. B. Koresko, and R. Poppen (1964). Stimulus generalization and the response-reinforcement contingency. J. exp. anal. Behav. 7:369-80.

Heise, G. A. and E. Boff (1962). Continuous avoidance as a base-line for measuring behavioral effects of drugs. Psychopharmacologia 3:264-82.

Hilgard, E. R. and G. H. Bower (1966). *Theories of Learning.* 3rd ed. New York: Appleton-Century Crofts.

Hill, R. T. (1970). Facilitation of conditioned reinforcement as a mechanism of psychomotor stimulation. In *Amphetamines and Related Compounds.* Proceedings of the Mario Negri Institute for Pharmacological Research, Milan, Italy. (E. Costa and S. Garattini, eds.). New York: Raven Press, pp. 781-95.

Hoffer, A. and H. Osmond (1967). *The Hallucinogens.* New York/London: Academic Press.

Hokfelt, T. and A. Ljungdahl (1972). Histochemie 29:325-39.

Holtz, W. C. and N. H. Azrin (1961). Discriminative properties of punishment. J. exp. anal. Behav. 4:225-32.

Holtzman, S. G. and J. E. Villarreal (1973). Operant behavior in the morphine-dependent rhesus monkey. J. Pharmac. exp. Ther. 184: 528-41.

Horn, G. and J. M. McKay (1973). Effects of lysergic acid diethylamide on the spontaneous activity and visual receptive fields of cells in the lateral geniculate nucleus of the cat. Exp. Brain Res. 17:271-84.

Hunt, H. F. and J. V. Brady (1955). Some effects of punishment and intercurrent "anxiety" on a simple operant. J. comp. physiol. Psychol. 48:305-10.

Hutchinson, R. R., N. H. Azrin, and G. M. Hunt (1968). Attack produced by intermittent reinforcement of a concurrent operant response. J. exp. anal. Behav. 11:489-95.

Hutchinson, R. R., N. H. Azrin, and J. W. Renfrew (1968). Effects of

References

shock intensity and duration on the frequency of biting attack by squirrel monkeys. J. exp. anal. Behav. 11:83-88.

Hutt, C. and S. J. Hutt (1965). Effects of environmental complexity on stereotyped behaviour of children. Ann. Behav. 13:1-4.

Iversen, L. L. (1967). *The Uptake and Storage of Noradrenaline in Sympathetic Nerves.* London: Cambridge University Press.

Iversen, L. L., ed. (1973). Catecholamines. Brit. Med. Bull. 29 (2):130-35.

Iversen, L. L. (1974). Monoamines in the central nervous system and the mode of action of antidepressant drugs. In *Biochemistry and Mental Illness.* (L. Iversen and S. Rose, eds.). London: Biochemical Society.

Iversen, S. D. and L. L. Iversen (1975). Chemical neurotransmitters and behavior. In *Textbook of Psychobiology.* (C. B. Blakemore and Gazzaniga, eds.). In press.

Janowsky, D. S., M. K. El-Yousel, J. M. Davis, and H. J. Sekerke (1973). Provocation of schizophrenic symptoms by intravenous methylphenidate. Arch. Gen. Psychiat. 28:185-91.

Janssen, P. A. J., C. J. E. Niemegeers, and K. H. L. Schellekens (1965). Is it possible to predict the clinical effects of neuroleptic drugs (major tranquillizers) from animal data? Part I. "Neuroleptic activity spectra" for rats. Arzneim-Forsch. 15:104-17.

Jarvik, M. E. and S. Chorover (1960). Impairment by lysergic acid diethylamide of accuracy in performance of a delayed alternation test in monkeys. Psychopharmacologia (Berl.) 1:221-30.

Jarvik, M. E. (1964). The influence of drugs upon memory. In *Animal Behavior and Drug Action.* (H. Steinberg, ed.). London: Churchill, pp. 44-60.

Jouvet, M. (1972). The role of monoamines and acetylcholine-containing neurons in the regulation of the sleep-waking cycle. Ergebn. der Physiol. 64:166-307.

Kelleher, R. T. and W. H. Morse (1964). Escape behavior and punished behavior. Fed. Proc. 23:808-17.

Kelleher, R. T. and W. H. Morse (1968). Determinants of the specificity of behavioral effects of drugs. Ergebn. der Physiol. 60:1-56.

Kelly, J. S. and L. P. Renaud (1973). Brit. J. Pharmac. 48:369-86.

Key, B. J. (1961). The effect of drugs on discrimination and sensory generalization of auditory stimuli in cats. Psychopharmacologia (Berl.) 2: 352-63.

Kimble, G. A. (1961). *Hilgard and Marquis Conditioning and Learning.* New York: Appleton-Century Crofts, Chapts. 3, 4.

Klein, D. F. and J. M. Davis (1969). *Diagnosis and Drug Treatment of Psychiatric Disorder.* Baltimore: Williams & Wilkins, pp. 52-138.

Klugh, H. E. and R. A. Patton (1959). Escape behavior of monkeys from

References

low intensity tone. Psychol. Rep. **5**:573-78.

Kriekhaus, E. E., N. E. Miller, and P. Zimmerman (1965). Reduction of freezing behavior and improvement of shock avoidance by d-amphetamine. J. comp. physiol. Psychol. **60**:36-40.

Krnjevic, C. (1975). In *Handbook of Psychopharmacology*. (L. Iversen, S. Iversen, and S. Snyder, eds.) vol. 2. New York: Plenum.

Kuhar, M. J., C. B. Pert, and S. H. Snyder (1973). Regional distribution of opiate receptor binding in monkey and human brain. Nature, **245**· 447-50.

Kulkarni, A. S. and W. M. Job (1967). Facilitation of avoidance learning by d-amphetamine. Life Sciences **6**:1579-87.

Kumar, R. (1969). Exploration and latent learning: Differential effects of dexamphetamine on components of exploratory behavior in rats. Psychopharmacologia (Berl.) **16**:54-72.

Larochelle, L., P. Bedard, L. J. Poirier, and T. L. Sourkes (1971). Correlative neuroanatomical and neuropharmacological study of tremor and catatonia in the monkey. Neuropharm. **10**:273-88.

Levine, S. (1962) The effects of infantile experience on adult behavior. *In Experimental Foundations of Clinical Psychology*. (A. J. Bachrach, ed.). New York: Basic Books.

Liddell, H. S. (1954). Conditioning and Emotions. Scient. Amer.

Livett, B. (1973). Brit. Med. Bull. **29**(2).

Lyon, M. and A. Randrup (1972). The dose-response effect of amphetamine upon avoidance behavior in the rat seen as a function of increasing stereotypy. Psychopharmacologia (Berl.) **23**:334-47.

McCleary, R. A. (1966). Response-modulating functions of the limbic system: Initiation and suppression. In *Progress in Physiological Psychology*. vol. 1. New York: Academic Press, pp. 209-272.

McKearney, J. W. (1968a). Maintenance of responding under a fixed interval schedule of electric shock presentation. Science **160**:1249-51.

McKearney, J. W. (1968b). The relative effects of d-amphetamine, imipramine and harmaline on tetrabenazine suppression of schedule-controlled behavior in the rat. J. Pharmac. exp. Ther. **159**:429-40.

McMillan, D. E. (1973a). Drugs and punished responding. I. Rate-dependent effects under multiple schedules. J. exp. anal. Behav. **19**: 133-45.

McMillan, D. E. (1973b). Drugs and punished responding. III. Punishment intensity as a determinant of drug effect. Psychopharmacologia (Berl.) **30**:61-74.

McMillan, D. E. and W. H. Morse (1967). Some effects of morphine and morphine antagonists on schedule-controlled behaviour. J. Pharmac. exp. Ther. **157**:175-84.

References

McMillan, D. E., L. S. Harris, J. M. Frankenhein, and J. S. Kennedy (1970). 1-Δ⁹-Trans-tetrahydrocannabinol in pigeons: Tolerance to the behavioral effects. Science 169:501-503.

Maffii, G. (1959). The secondary conditioned response of rats and the effects of some psychopharmacological agents. J. Pharmac. Pharmacol. 11:129-39.

Maier, N. R. F. (1949). *Frustration: The Study of Behavior without a Goal.* New York: McGraw-Hill.

Malmo, R. B. (1959). Activation: A neuropsychological dimension. Psychol. Rev. 66:367-86.

Marchbanks, R. (1975). In *Handbook of Psychopharmacology.* (L. Iversen, S. Iversen, and S. Snyder, eds.), vol. I. New York: Plenum.

Masserman, J. H. (1943). *Behavior and Neurosis.* Chicago: University of Chicago Press.

Masserman, J. H. and C. Pechtel (1956). An experimental investigation of factors influencing drug action. Psychiat. Res. Rep. 95-113.

Mello,, N. K. and J. H. Mendelson (1972). Drinking patterns during work-contingent and non-contingent alcohol acquisition. Psychosom. Med. 34:139-64.

Miczek, K. A. (1973). Effects of scopolamine, amphetamine and chlordiazepoxide on punishment. Psychopharmacologia (Berl.) 28:373-89.

Miller, N. E. and Carmona, A. (1967) Modification of a visceral response, salivation in thirsty dogs, by instrumental training with water reward. J. comp. physiol. Psychol. 63:1-6.

Miller, N. E. and L. DiCara (1967). Instrumental learning of heart rate changes in curarized rats: Shaping, and specificity to discriminate stimulus. J. comp. physiol. Psych. 63:12-19.

Miller, R. J. and C. R. Hiley (1974). Anti-muscarinic properties of neuroleptics and drug induced parkinsonism. Nature 248:596-97.

Morse, W. H. (1962). Use of operant conditioning, techniques for evaluating the effects of barbiturates on behavior. In *First Habnemann Symposium on Psychosomatic Medicine.* New York: Lea & Febiger, pp. 275-81.

Morse, W. H. (1964). Effects of amobarbital and chlorpromazine on punished behaviour in the pigeon. Psychopharmacologia (Berl.) 6:286-94.

Mowrer, O. H. (1939) A stimulus-response analysis of anxiety and its role as a reinforcing agent. Psychol. Rev. 46:553-65.

Myer, J. S. (1966). Punishment of instinctive behavior: Suppression of mouse-killing by rats. Psychon. Sci. 4:385-86.

Myer, J. S. (1968). Associative and temporal determinants of facilitation and inhibition of attack by pain. J. comp. physiol. Psychol. 66:17-21.

Myer, J. S. and D. Ricci (1968). Delay of punishment for the goldfish. J.

References

comp. physiol. Psychol. **66**:417-21.

O'Kelly, L. I. and L. C. Steckle (1939). A note on long-enduring emotional responses in the rat. J. Psychol. **8**:125-31.

Oliverio, A. (1968). Effects of scopolamine on avoidance conditioning and habituation of mice. Psychopharmacologia (Berl.) **12**:214-26.

Olson, L. and Fuxe, K. (1972). Further mapping out of central noradrenaline neuron systems: Projections of the subcoeruleus area. Brain Res. **43**:289-95.

Overton, D. A. (1966). State-dependent learning produced by depressant and atropine-like drugs. Psychopharmacologia (Berl.) **10**:6-31.

Pappas, G. D. and S. T. G. Waxman (1972). In *Structure and Function of Synapses*. (G. D. Pappas and D. P. Purpura, eds.) New York: Raven Press. p. 11.

Peters, A. (1970). In *Contemporary Research Methods in Neuroanatomy*. (W. J. H. Nauta and S. O. E. Ebbesson, eds.). New York: Springer-Verlag, p. 65.

Poschel, B. P. H. and F. W. Ninteman (1963). Norepinephrine: A possible excitatory neurohormone of the reward system. Life Sciences **3**:782-88.

Randrup, A. and I. Munkvad (1970). Biochemical, anatomical and psychological investigations of stereotyped behavior induced by amphetamines. In *Amphetamines and Related Compounds*. (E. Costa and S. Garratini, eds.). New York: Raven Press, pp. 695-713.

Ray, D. S. (1972). *Drugs, Society and Human Behavior*. St. Louis: Mosby.

Rech, R. H. (1965). Amphetamine effects on poor performance of rats in a shuttle-box. Psychopharmacologie (Berl.) **9**:110-17.

Rech, R. H. and K. E. Moore (1971). *An Introduction to Psychopharmacology*. New York: Raven Press, p. 99.

Revusky, S. H. (1968). Aversion to sucrose produced by contingent x-irradiation: Temporal and dosage parameters. J. comp. physiol. Psychol. **65**:17-22.

Reynolds, G. S. (1968). *A Primer of Operant Conditioning*. Glenview (Ill.): Scott Foresman.

Robbins, T. and S. D. Iversen (1973). A dissociation of the effects of d-amphetamine on locomotor activity and exploration in rats. Psychopharmacologia (Berl.) **28**:155-64.

Rushton, R. and H. Steinberg (1964). Modification of behavioural effects of drugs by past experience. In *Animal Behaviour and Drug Action*. (H. Steinberg, ed.). London: Churchill, pp. 207-18.

Rutledge, C. O. and R. T. Kelleher (1965). Interactions between the effects of methamphetamine and pentobarbital on operant behavior in the pigeon. Psychopharmacologia (Berl.) **7**:400-408.

References

Schachter, S. and J. E. Singer (1962). Cognitive, social and physiological determinants of emotional state. Psychol. Rev. **69**:379-99.

Scheckel, C. L. (1965). Self-adjustment of the interval in delayed matching: Limit of delay for the rhesus monkey. J. comp. physiol. Psychol. **59**:415-18.

Scheckel, C. L., Boff, E., Dahlen, P. and Smart, T. (1968). Behavioral effects in monkeys of racemates of two biologically active marijuana constituents. Science **160**:1467-69.

Schildkraut, J. J. (1965). The catecholamine hypothesis of affective disorders: A review of supporting evidence. Am. J. Psychiat. **122**:509-22.

Schiørring, E. (1971). Amphetamine-induced selective stimulation of certain items with concurrent inhibition of others in an open-field test with rats. Behaviour **39**:1-17.

Schiørring, E. and A. Hecht (1900). Behavioural responses of non-tolerant rat groups to the administration of 2mg/kg morphine in an open-field test. (In preparation.)

Schopler, E. (1965). Early infantile autism and receptor processes. Arch. Gen. Psychiat. **13**:327-35.

Schou, M. (1963). Normothymotics, "mood-normalizers." Are lithium and imipramine drugs specific for affective disorders. Brit. J. Psychiat. **109**: 803-809.

Schuster, C. R. and J. H. Woods (1968). The conditioned reinforcing effects of stimuli associated with morphine reinforcement. Int. J. Addictions, **3**:223-30.

Shapiro, M. M. (1961). Salivary conditioning in dogs during fixed-interval reinforcement contingent upon lever pressing. J. exp. anal. Behav. **4**: 361-64.

Shute, C. C. D. and P. R. Lewis (1967). The ascending cholinergic reticular systems: Neocortical, olfactory and subcortical projections. Brain **90**:487-520.

Sidman, M. (1956). Drug-behavior interaction. Ann. N.Y. Acad. Sci. **65**: 282-302.

Sidman, M. (1960). Normal sources of pathological behavior. Science **132**: 61-68.

Silverman, A. P. (1965). Ethological and statistical analysis of drug effects on the social behaviour of laboratory rats. Brit. J. Pharmac. **24**: 579-90.

Smythies, J. R., R. J. Bradley, V. S. Johnston, and F. Leonard (1967). The behavioural effects of some derivatives of mescaline and N,N-dimethyltryptamine in the rat. Life Sciences **6**:1887-93.

Snyder, S. H., E. Richelson, H. Weingaftner, and L. A. Faillace (1970). Psychotropic methoxyamphetamines: Structure and activity in man.

References

In *Amphetamines and Related Compounds.* (E. Costa and S. Garrattini, eds.). New York: Raven Press, pp. 905-28.

Snyder, S. H. (1974). Catecholamines as mediators of drug effects in schizophrenia. In *Neurosciences: Third Study Program.* (F. O. Schmitt and F. Worden, eds.). Cambridge (Mass.): MIT Press, pp. 721-32.

Solomon, R. L. (1964). Punishment. Amer. Psychol. **19**:239-53.

Stein, L. (1968) Chemistry of reward and punishment. In *Psychopharmacology: A Review of Program, 1957-1967.* (D. H. Efron, ed.). Washington, D.C.: U.S. Government Printing Office.

Stein, L. and C. D. Wise (1969). Release of norepinephrine from hypothalamus and amygdala by rewarding medial forebrain bundle stimulation and amphetamine. J. comp. physiol. Psychol. **67**:189-98.

Stein, L., C. D. Wise, and B. D. Berger (1973). Antianxiety action of benzodiazepines: Decrease in activity of serotonin neurons in the punishment system. In *The Benzodiazepines.* New York: Raven Press, pp. 299-326.

Stretch, R. and G. J. Gerber (1973). Drug-induced reinstatement of amphetamine self-administration behaviour in monkeys. Canad. J. Psychol. **27**:168-79.

Summerfield, A. (1964). Drugs and human behaviour. Brit. Med. Bull. **20**: 70-74.

Taylor, K. M. and S. H. Snyder (1971). Differential effects of D- and L-amphetamine on behavior and on catecholamine disposition in dopamine and noradrenaline containing neurons of rat brain. Brain Res. **28**:295-309.

Terrace, H. S. (1963). Errorless discrimination learning in the pigeon: Effects of chlorpromazine and imipramine. Science **140**:318-19.

Thompson, J. and C. R. Schuster (1964). Morphine self-administration food-reinforced and avoidance behaviour in rhesus monkeys. Psychopharmocologia (Berl.) **5**:87-94.

Thompson, T. and C. R. Schuster (1968). *Behavioral Pharmacology.* New York: Prentice-Hall.

Thompson, T. and R. Pickens (1971). Drugs as reinforcers: Schedules condiderations. In *Symposium on Schedules Influence and Behavioral Pharmacology.* (R. Gilbert, ed.). New York: Academic Press, pp. 50-64.

Ullman, A. D. (1951). The experimental production and analysis of a "compulsive eating symptom" in rats. J. comp. physiol. Psychol. **44**: 575-81.

Ulrich, R. E., R. R. Hutchinson, and N. H. Azrin (1965). Pain-elicited aggression. Psychol. Rec. **15**:111-26.

References

Ungerstedt, U., L. L. Butcher, S. G. Butcher, N-E Anden, and K. Fuxe (1969). Direct chemical stimulation of dopaminergic mechanisms in the neostriatum of the rat. Brain Res. 14:461-71.

Ungerstedt, U. (1971). On the anatomy, pharmacology and function of the nigro-striatal dopamine system. Acta. physiol. Scand. Suppl. 367.

Usdin, E. and S. H. Snyder, eds. (1974). *Frontiers in Catecholamine Research.* Oxford: Pergamon Press.

Vaillant, G. E. (1964). A comparison of chlorpromazine and imipramine on behaviour of the pigeon. J. Pharmac. exp. Ther. 146:377-84.

Verhave, T., J. E. Owen, and E. B. Robbins (1959). The effect of morphine sulphate on avoidance and escape behaviour. J. Pharmac. exp. Ther. 125:248-57.

Wade, M. (1947). The effect of sedatives upon delayed response in monkeys following removal of the prefrontal lobes. J. Neurophysiol. 10: 57-61.

Warburton, D. M. (1972). The cholinergic control of internal inhibition. In *Inhibition and Learning.* (R. Boakes and M. S. Halliday, eds.). London: Academic Press, pp. 431-60.

Weiss, B. (1956). The effects of various morphine-N-allyl-normorphine ratios on behaviour. Arch. intern. Pharacodynamie Therap. 105:381-88.

Weiss, B. and A. Heller (1969). Methodological problems in evaluating the role of cholinergic mechanisms in behavior. Fed. Proc. 28:135-46.

Weiss, B. and V. G. Laties (1958). Fractional escape and avoidance on a titration schedule. Science 128:1575-76.

Weiss, B. and V. G. Laties (1961). Behavioral thermoregulation. Science 133:1338-44.

Weiss, B. and V. G. Laties (1964a). Drug effects on the temporal patterning of behavior. Fed. Proc. 23:801-807.

Weiss, B. and V. G. Laties (1964b). Analgesic effects on monkeys of morphine nalorphine and a benzomorphan narcotic antagonist. J. Pharmac. exp. Ther. 143:169-73.

Weiss, J. M., E. E. Krieckhaus, and R. Conte (1968). Effects of fear conditioning on subsequent avoidance behaviour and movement. J. comp. physiol. psychol. 65:413-21.

Weissman, A. (1959). Differential drug effects upon a three-ply multiple schedule of reinforcement. J. exp. anal. Behav. 2:271-87.

Weiskrantz, L., C. G. Gross, and V. Baltzer (1965). The beneficial effects of meprobramate on delayed response performance in the frontal monkey. Quart. J. exp. Psychol. 17:118-24.

Weiskrantz, L. (1968). Emotion. In *Analysis of Behavioral Change.* (L. Weiskrantz, ed.). New York: Harper & Row, pp. 50-90.

References

Wenzel, B. M. (1959). Relative resistance to reserpine of responses based on positive, as compared with negative, reinforcement. J. comp. physiol. Psychol. **52**:673-81.

Wikler, A. (1965). Conditioning factors in opiate addiction and relapse. In *Narcotics*. (D. M. Wilner & G. G. Kassebaum, eds). New York: McGraw-Hill, pp. 85-100.

Winger, G. D. and J. H. Woods (1973). The reinforcing property of ethanol in the rhesus monkey: I. Initiation, maintenance and termination of intravenous ethanol-reinforced responding. Ann. N.Y. Acad. Sci. **215**:162-75.

Wikler, A. and F. T. Pescor (1963). Classical conditioning of a morphine abstinence phenomenon, reinforcement of opiod-drinking behaviour and relapse in morphine-addicted rats. Psychopharmacologia (Berl.) **10**:235-84.

Wise, C. D. and L. Stein (1969). Facilitation of brain self-stimulation by central administration of norepinephrine. Science **163**:299-301.

Wuttke, W. and R. T. Kelleher (1970). Effects of some benzodiazepines on punished and unpunished behaviour in the pigeon. (1970) J. Pharmac. exp. Ther. **172**:397-405.

Yamamura, H. I. and S. H. Snyder (1973). High affinity transport of choline into synaptosomes of rat brain. J. Neurochem. **21**:1355-74.

York, D. (1975). In *Handbook of Psychopharmacology*. (L. Iversen, S. Iversen, and S. Snyder, eds.). New York: Plenum.

Zbinden, G. and Randall, L. O. (1967). Pharmacology of Benzodiazepines: Laboratory and clinical correlations. Adv. Pharm. **5**:213-91.

Index

Acetylcholine, and agonist and antagonist drugs, 103–8; distribution in CNS pathways, 133–36; drug effects on metabolism, 100–3; neurotransmitter role of, 81, 82
Acetylcholinesterase, 101–3, 133, 134
Acetyl-β-methylcholine, 104
Aggression, shock induced, 41–42
Agonist drugs, 61
Amitriptyline, 196, 197
Amphetamines, in combination with barbiturates, 183; dose-response curves for d- and l-isomers, 63; effect on behavior reinforced by food or shock avoidance, 146; effect on nigral cell firing, 92; effects on behavior, 170–79; neuropharmacology of, 167–70; psychosis with, 269–75; structure of, 110
Analgesics, behavioral dissociation of morphine and barbiturate, 161–63
Antidepressant drugs, behavioral characterization of, 164–65; behavioral effects of, 199–204; dissociation from phenothiazines, 199–201; and neurochemical theories of affective disorders, 282–86; neuropharmacology of, 193–98
Antagonist drugs, 61

Apomorphine, as agonist at DA receptors, 117; effect on nigral cell firing, 92; effects of neuroleptic drugs and, 275, 276
Arecoline, 104
Arousal, effects of barbiturates, 180; effects of stimulants, 170–72
Atropine, effects of EEG, 90; effects on learning and memory, 190, 191; as muscarinic antagonist, 104, 105
Aversive stimuli, and change in schedule of reinforcement, 52–54; extinction of, 49; novelty, 46–48; poison as, 33–34; and shock, 26–31; shock threshold and effects of opiates, 210–14

Barbiturates, as anti-anxiety drugs, 223, 228–29; effects on behavior, 180–83; hepatic metabolism of, 74; neuropharmacology of, 179, 180; penetration into the cerebrospinal fluid, 69
Batrochotoxin, 89
Benzodiazepines, 223–37; effect on immediate punishment, 229–31
Benztropine, 104, 105, 114
Bicuculline, 95, 124, 125
Blood-brain barrier, 65–70
Butyrophenones. See Neuroleptic drugs

Index

Index